Anatomy of
a Psychiatric Illness

Healing the Mind
and the Brain

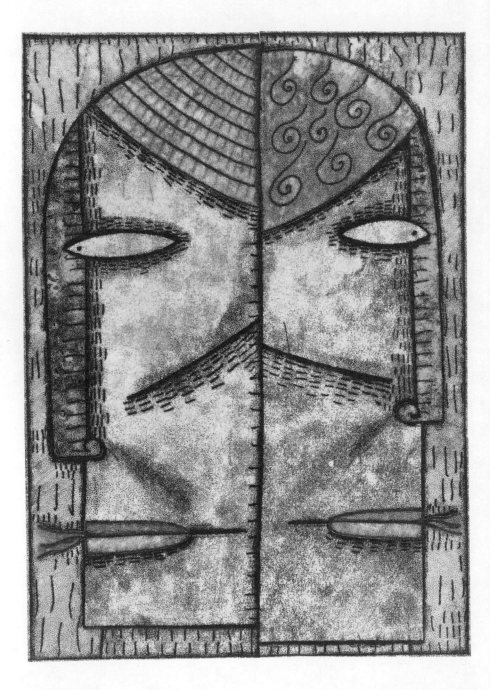

Anatomy of a Psychiatric Illness

Healing the Mind and the Brain

Keith Russell Ablow, M.D.

Foreword by
George D. Lundberg, M.D.

Illustrations by Richard Downs

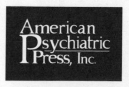

American Psychiatric Press, Inc.

Washington, DC
London, England

Copyright © 1993   Keith Russell Ablow
ALL RIGHTS RESERVED
Manufactured in the United States of America on acid-free paper
97 96 95 94   4 3 2 1
First Edition

American Psychiatric Press, Inc.
1400 K Street, N.W., Washington, DC   20005

Library of Congress Cataloging-in-Publication Data
Ablow, Keith R.
   Anatomy of a psychiatric illness :   healing the mind and the brain / Keith Russell Ablow. — 1st ed.
      p.   cm.
   Includes bibliographical references and index.
   ISBN 0-88048-521-3 (alk. paper)
   1. Psychiatry—Popular works. 2. Psychiatry—Philosophy. 3. Mental illness—Case studies. I. Title.
   [DNLM: 1. Mental Disorders—case studies. 2. Psychotherapy—case studies. WM 40 A152a 1993]
   RC460.A23 1993
   616.89—dc20
   DNLM/DLC   93-13483
   for Library of Congress   CIP

British Library Cataloguing in Publication Data
A CIP record is available from the British Library.

This book is dedicated to Gary Goldstein and Deborah Small.
What joy it has been to never be without a friend.

As a psychiatrist, I run into a major difficulty at the outset: how can I go straight to the patients if the psychiatric words at my disposal keep the patient at a distance from me? How can one demonstrate the general human relevance and significance of the patient's condition if the words one has to use are specifically designed to isolate and circumscribe the meaning of the patient's life to a particular clinical entity?

—R. D. Laing

Contents

Thinking About the Mind

Thinking About Society

Acknowledgments

No book is the author's alone. This one has grown directly from my relationships with patients. It is by sitting with them—listening to the stories of their illnesses—that I learned that the lessons of neuropharmacology and neuroanatomy could not fully explain psychiatric suffering, much less fully heal it.

I am also grateful to Dr. George Lundberg for providing the foreword to this book. I, like countless other physician-writers and physician-editors, have been inspired by his example.

In Richard Downs I have found a rare artist who can translate written themes and thoughts into images that enrich my work.

Finally, I thank Dr. Carol Nadelson, Ron McMillen, Claire Reinburg, Pam Harley, Greg Kuny, Belinda Josey, Pam Maher, Joanie Lefkowitz, Jon Jensen, and Maria Lavorata of the American Psychiatric Press. This is their book as well.

Foreword

When I was on the faculty of the University of Southern California School of Medicine in the 1970s, they created a basic sciences group call the Department of Behavioral Sciences. As a pathologist and toxicologist, I ridiculed that decision, saying that human behavior was not a science, that it probably wasn't even an art.

Fortunately, that embarrassingly pejorative bias I felt and expressed is long gone. My respect for the neurosciences now grows by the day as I see solid article after solid article in this field sent to our general medical journal, JAMA, to be handled by our deputy editor, Dr. Richard Glass, himself a highly regarded psychiatrist. And, as I observe the emergence of biological psychiatry and psychopharmacology, and now even the molecular genetics of psychiatric illnesses, on the pages of our *Archives of General Psychiatry*, so skillfully shepherded there by the redoubtable Daniel X. Freedman for these past seventeen years, I become even more impressed.

But, there is oh so much more to learn. When we hear that 20 percent of all Americans have one or more episodes of diagnosable psychiatric illness or substance addiction each year; when interpersonal violence of all kinds in our population seems at record heights; and when around 140 armed conflicts (somewhat short of war) are going on in the world in 1993, we as humans must worry about neurosciences and human behavior as a highest priority.

Millennia ago, we learned how to prevent hunger and treat starvation—it's called food. Yet, in this century, after we have learned how to farm to overabundance, hundreds of millions of people go hungry every day, and malnutrition—even fatal starvation—is common in much of the Third World. Why? Flaws in human behavior. Is it a psychiatric illness? I don't know which one to call it (by DSM-III-R), but it certainly isn't mental health. Defects in human behavior always have been the bane of human existence. After all, what are the age-old enemies of physicians? They are premature death, disability, disease, pain, human suffering. Everything else is nothing but noise.

I first met the author, Dr. Keith Ablow, several years ago when he was a medical student at Johns Hopkins University. He was working on the medical student section of JAMA called PULSE and was obviously very interested and skillful in communicating medical information to medical students. He was asked to head up a strategic planning effort for PULSE, which at that time was a newsletter that was inserted into only those copies of JAMA distributed to medical students. While the regular United States JAMA circulation was about 350,000, that to medical students was only about 35,000—the student members of the American Medical Association. Keith was challenged to consider what it would take to upgrade the brief newsletter's quality, size, consistency, and predictability so that it would merit being placed in the regular JAMA once a month. All doctors and libraries throughout the world could then receive it, read it, benefit from it and keep it.

Keith Ablow did exactly that. Working with other students, he devised a strategic plan, set objectives, determined necessary actions, set up a budget and a timetable and determined who was responsible for what. I implemented his plan promptly. It continues to be followed, still allowing us to train blossoming medical editors and writers as students, in addition to providing information to all doctors from the student's viewpoint. Quite a lasting feat for former medical student Ablow.

Later, I ran into Keith in television studios in Hollywood and New York when he was on elective from school expanding his learning into television journalism by working on the job.

Back to this book. What in the realm of potential human experience could be more interesting than the inside and inside-out workings of the human brain and the human mind? I believe nothing. And this remarkably readable book about so many facets of the human mind—thinking, feeling, behaving—and the various interwoven misfires portrays a cornucopia of psychiatric knowledge, vividly illustrated by example after example of the inside-out of real human experiences.

If you like people and their foibles at all, you will love this book.

George D. Lundberg, M.D.
Editor, JAMA

Preface

> The poets and philosophers before me discovered the unconscious;
> what I discovered was the scientific method by which the unconscious
> can be studied.
>
> —Sigmund Freud 1926

Psychiatrists are, in some ways, guests in the house of medicine. We
are not the same as other doctors. We know we are different,
patients know it, and our colleagues sense it, too. No medical specialists
inspire in the profession and the community a more dramatic mixture of
respect, fear, and ridicule.

Those who have not needed our services personally, nor sought them
for a loved one, often have little understanding of what we do. The
psychiatrist's public image remains a collage of media stereotypes gar-
nered from movies such as *One Flew Over the Cuckoo's Nest* and *Ordi-
nary People*.

We provoke questions that are not put to internists, cardiologists or
endocrinologists. How much are we scientists and how much philoso-
phers? Do we treat disease or depravity? Are we agents for personal
freedom or social control? Do our medicines cure illnesses or merely
quell emotions? Is what we do effective or futile?

As psychiatrists, we silently struggle with these questions ourselves.
In less than 100 years, our field has stretched its conceptual base from
the ego and id all the way to neurotransmitters and positron-emission
tomography. Our repertoire of perspectives on psychiatric illness has
expanded to the point that the same psychiatrist may understand depression in one individual as anger turned upon the self, and depression

in another person as the result of a stroke destroying nerve cells in the left frontal lobe of the brain. We are called upon to be expert in psychotherapies that treat the mind and in pharmacologies that treat the brain.

We take as our domain not only the suffering of those with major mental illnesses such as schizophrenia, not only the pain of those scarred by tragedy or misfortune, but even the lost possibilities of those living life at the mercy of unconscious conflicts.

We are the front line in containing violence in the emergency room, the experts called to assess a patient's competency to refuse medical treatment, the empathic ear to those facing debilitating physical illness, the primary caretakers of the chronically psychotic and the transiently disturbed, champions of the examined life.

We are faced with issues that transcend biology and anatomy and challenge us to think about the nature of humanity. We wonder, for instance, whether pervasive character flaws in an individual should be thought of as illness, rather than meanspiritedness or evil. We ponder the connection between creativity and some forms of mental illness. We debate whether there can be rational suicide. We have strong beliefs about the conditions under which an individual should be relieved of responsibility for his or her actions.

These issues emerge against a backdrop of burgeoning technology, ever-increasing financial constraints and an expanded role for the law in medicine.

Yet for a field grappling vigorously with questions that cut to the core of human existence, we are a quiet profession. The ways we think about behavior and emotion are so intricately woven and often so deeply held that they have become something of a private trust.

A young woman I treat for depression and drug addiction recently stopped relating her story midsentence. She looked inquisitively at me taking notes.

"Yes?" I asked.

"I'd just love to know what you're thinking when you're listening to patients," she said. "How do you put it all together?"

This book is the shortest answer I dare give. After reading the chapters that follow, you, the reader, will understand not only the symptoms of many psychiatric conditions, but some of the ways psychiatrists elicit, categorize and treat those symptoms. You will join the struggle to blend chemistry and compassion, philosophy and physiology, in proper measure. You will begin, perhaps, to grasp the frustrations and exhilarations of those who are working in a profession with roots in morality and ethics and towering branches into the neurosciences.

Most of all, I hope that you take the time between paragraphs and pages—as I have between patients—to reflect on the wonderful, if sometimes painful, diversity of human experience and on psychiatry's remarkable potential to relieve human suffering.

Thinking
About Patients

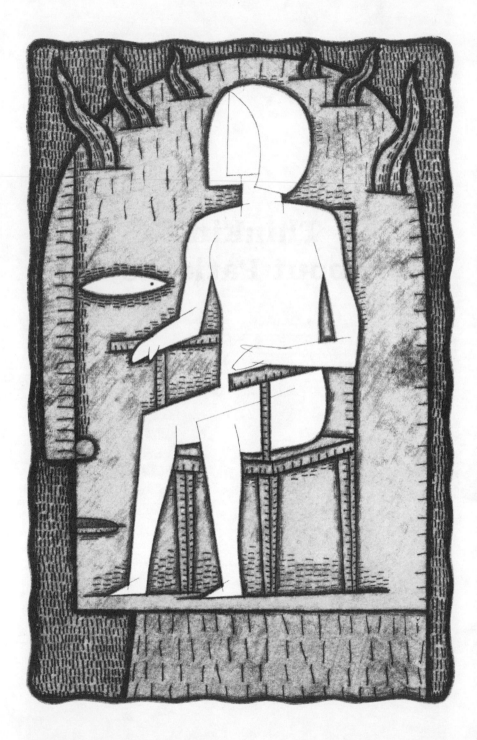

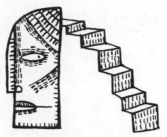

The Man Who Lost His Family

Oliver was panicked when he first came to see me at the hospital's outpatient clinic. He had a long and frightening story to tell, and no one seemed willing to listen—not the governor's office, not the FBI, not even the CIA. He was sure that the staffers who always dismissed him after just a few minutes of his explanation were either incompetent or deceitful.

He was forty-three years old, but looked older. He wore overalls with a bright red bandana tucked in one pocket.

Dark lenses covered his eyes. He moved his chair to the corner of the room furthest from me before sitting down.

"I've come here because I don't know how else to handle the pressure I'm under," he said.

"What pressure is that?" I asked.

"My daughter's been kidnapped," he muttered, beginning to cry. "She's gone. And no one is doing anything to find her."

He took a sheet of paper out of one pocket. It was a letter, written in a hurried hand, addressed to several city officials. In it, Oliver described his horror at having discovered that his daughter had been replaced by a

---

Portions of this chapter were first published in *The Washington Post*.

masquerading double, a nearly perfect copy whose physical differences were so slight that only a parent could detect them. To him it was obvious, however, that his real daughter's hair was finer than that of the girl who now claimed her place. And his real daughter's nose had been angled slightly more to the right.

"How long have you known she was gone?" I asked.

"A month," he said. "A month of pure hell. I've looked everywhere. Asked everyone. I'm so confused at this point I can't think where to turn." He glared at me. "You'll want to throw medicines at me. Well, I don't need 'em. I don't. I need someone to listen to me, for Christ's sake!"

I sat with him as he sobbed. "Can we go over this from the beginning?" I asked. "I need to know when things started to go wrong in your life."

"I'm not here for medicines," he warned, again. "And I'm not going in any hospital. I've been through that at another clinic. I just walked right out."

"I don't think we should consider medicine until we've talked," I assured him. "I want to understand what has happened to you."

The set of symptoms with which Oliver was suffering has been called *Capgras' syndrome*, named for the French psychiatrist Jean Marie Joseph Capgras (1873–1950). The main sign of this syndrome is the patient's false and unshakable belief (called a *delusion*) that other individuals in his or her life are not their real selves, but imposters, often with evil intent.

Capgras' syndrome is generally the hallmark of an underlying major mental illness such as schizophrenia or an affective (mood) disorder such as depression. Some researchers have suggested that a blow to the head or a stroke affecting the right side of the brain may cause it, as well.

Whatever its roots, the personal impact of the syndrome on Oliver was devastating. He wholeheartedly believed that his daughter had been taken from him. She could have been tortured. She might or might not still be alive. What's more, his efforts to enlist others in his search for her had been in vain. Police officers had mocked him. Neighbors were shunning him. How far, he wondered, could the conspiracy reach? Was anyone to be trusted? He felt utterly alone against an awesome enemy— one capable of assuming any human form it chose. The world had become a hostile place.

My first concern was to keep Oliver safe. I questioned him repeatedly about his potential for violence. Did he plan to attack the imposter? Was he so discouraged that he would take his own life? He assured me that his plan was to peacefully resolve this bizarre drama.

Knowing that Oliver had left another clinic as soon as medication was suggested, I felt that my only chance to be helpful was to be the empathic ear he had requested. I needed to ally with the person *behind* the illness, to listen to his pain and begin to understand the terror he felt.

In several hour-long sessions I began piecing together Oliver's history. His memories of his own childhood varied from cloudy to frankly psychotic. He insisted, for example, that he had been literally "thrown in the trash" as a fetus, then rescued and passed from foster home to foster home. The foster parents had been famous movie stars and politicians, such as Elizabeth Taylor, Marilyn Monroe and John Kennedy. He had more credible memories of severe beatings and sexual abuse, though he was unsure at whose hand. He seemed to have lost his memory for whole segments of his life.

The assertion that he had been raised by celebrities made me more suspicious that Oliver's underlying illness might be mania, an illness of mood in which patients often have increased energy, decreased need for sleep and grandiose ideas. Patients with mania can indeed develop delusions about being involved in elaborate plots. And whereas many manic individuals feel euphoric, others feel irritable.

Oliver did tell me that he needed far less sleep than before. He also reported another symptom of mania—the sense that thoughts were *racing* through his head.

Medical records from the Massachusetts state hospital system shed more light on his story. His father had become depressed in his thirties and required a psychiatric hospitalization. Over the next several years, he was admitted four more times. At least once, he showed the increased energy and grandiosity typical of mania.

Oliver's mother was an alcoholic who physically abused her son, resulting in the foster home placements he now barely recalled.

Even with his chaotic childhood, Oliver had apparently gone on to graduate from high school and college. He brought me letters of recommendation from very responsible jobs he had held, some as recently as four years before. They were positions that required quick thinking and superior organizational skills.

After achieving so much, something had abruptly gone wrong. I wondered whether the sudden change in his life might have been due to the beginnings in him of the mental illness that had affected his father. Alternatively, he could have become addicted to substances, as had his mother. He might even have suffered a physical illness—such as a stroke or a central nervous system infection—that could account for his current psychiatric symptoms.

"What went wrong that you stopped working four years ago?" I asked.

"My wife died," he said immediately. "Hit by a car. Right out of the blue. I haven't been the same since. I don't eat right. I don't sleep."

"What was she like?"

He took a deep breath. "What was she *like?* She was a knowing woman. She had a sixth sense about people. She was a beautiful person."

I nodded.

"I cried once," he said. "I cried and I threw up. If I start to cry now, I won't ever stop." He looked away from me.

I felt that the core around which Oliver's suffering revolved had been uncovered. "Nothing in your life seems to be permanent," I said quietly.

He took off his dark glasses for the first time in weeks, revealing bright blue eyes. "This girl who claims to be my daughter," he said, "is always talking about moving to California."

"And how does that make you feel?" I asked.

"It's a dead giveaway," he said. "My daughter wouldn't be telling me these things. This one's all grown up like a woman, not a girl."

It made intuitive sense to me that with Oliver's chaotic childhood, including a very sick father and an addicted mother, the abrupt loss of his stable marriage could have precipitated his illness. When his daughter then revealed plans to move away, it may have been too much for him to bear. She was maturing to a young woman, and her impending departure from him (both physically and emotionally) was all mixed up with unresolved grief over his wife's death. Unable to focus feelings of anger and abandonment on someone he cared so much about, his mind had actually substituted an evil double to despise.

"Who do you have to rely on in your life?" I asked.

"You want to know something, honestly?" he asked.

I nodded.

"Not a soul. Do you know my daughter and I sat alone by my wife's bed in the intensive care unit for four days? Alone, waiting for her to die. And not one friend came by. Not a single one of my relatives." He squinted at me, looking me over from head to toe.

"Are you troubled by something you see over here?" I asked.

"I can't even tell if *you're* real," he said. He leaned toward me, then got up from his seat and started over to mine.

Although I felt uneasy, I stayed seated.

He stopped within a few feet and gently touched my shoulder with one finger. He exerted a bit more pressure. I didn't move. He gripped my biceps. Then he let go, walked back to his seat and slowly sat down, looking relieved.

"You seem solid enough," he said. "I wasn't sure for a second. The light was hitting you funny."

I understood Oliver's doubt about my physical presence as an expression of his fear that I, like his mother, father, friends and, now, his daughter, would abandon him. "I'm here," I said. "I care about what's happened to you."

"You have plans to move?" he asked, without the slightest trace of humor.

"I plan to be here for a long time," I said.

With that, Oliver began to cry. I believe he sensed that I understood some of his fear of death and separation and isolation.

It was true that sitting with Oliver had, from the beginning of our work together, unearthed my own fears. Several times during our sessions I felt the emptiness in my stomach that I used to feel when preparing to leave home for nursery school and first grade. My dogged refusal to attend, in fact, interrupted my early education. Many psychiatrists believe that the kind of school phobia I experienced stems from a child's anxiety that a tragedy during the day will claim his or her loved ones.

There were other memories coming to me. I recalled the sense of impending doom I felt when a boyhood friend was diagnosed with cancer. My mind wandered to the night I had visited a close colleague of mine who, like Oliver's wife, had been hit by a car and was dying in an intensive care unit.

The trust developing between us not only allowed Oliver to begin sharing his grief with me, but also gave me the chance to obtain medical information about him that he had been reticent to reveal earlier on. This was very important data because I knew that the emotional dynamics that seemed to be such a powerful explanation of his symptoms were only one way to understand his condition. Bodily abnormalities, such as thyroid disease, brain injury and even cancer, can also cause psychotic thinking.

Although there was nothing in Oliver's medical history that was of particular concern, I told him I needed to have his blood tested and to order other tests, such as a CAT scan of his head.

"You think I'm crazy, don't you?" he said, accusingly. "You don't believe my daughter's been kidnapped at all."

"You've been under tremendous stress," I said evenly. "You've lost something precious. I want to make sure you haven't become physically ill, as well."

Oliver reluctantly consented. I referred him to an internist who performed a comprehensive physical examination, sent Oliver's blood for analysis and ordered a CAT scan. The results were all normal.

Over the next weeks we began to do the work of grieving that Oliver had left undone after his wife's sudden death. We spoke of their courtship, their honeymoon, the challenges of their first year of marriage, the birth of their daughter. At times, Oliver seemed overwhelmed by nearly unbearable sadness; at other times, he would smile and laugh at touching memories of his wife.

"I've been paying the price for not letting myself grieve, haven't I?" he asked once.

"I think that's right," I said.

His delusion about his daughter's kidnapping, never far from center stage, reasserted itself. "It's going to get in the way of finding my daughter's kidnappers," he said. "It's going to prevent me from thinking clearly about how to get her back."

I felt Oliver and I had established enough trust so that I could recommend medication without destroying our alliance. "I think medication might make it easier for you to organize your thoughts," I told him. "I've gotten to know you. I know that medicine could be very helpful."

"I don't like medicines," he said. He shifted in his chair. "Who would prescribe it, anyway?"

"I would," I said.

"You? You wouldn't be referring me somewhere else?"

I shook my head.

"I don't go for medicines. I'll think about it, but the whole idea . . . Just let me think about it."

It took two more weeks for Oliver to agree to try the antipsychotic medication haloperidol. Haloperidol is thought to work by blunting the action of a chemical messenger in the brain, called dopamine, over-activity of which has been linked to psychotic disorders such as mania.

A week after starting haloperidol, Oliver began to doubt that the girl living in his house could be an imposter.

"She's an incredible copy," he said. He shook his head and let his breath out slowly. "Is it possible" he asked, beginning to cry, "that I'm going to miss her so much that she just seems to be gone?"

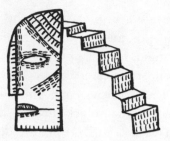

2

Classrooms, Cadavers, Compassion and the Soul

"Maybe the knowledge is too great and maybe men are growing too small," said Lee. "Maybe, kneeling down to atoms, they're becoming atom-sized in their souls. Maybe a specialist is only a coward, afraid to look out of his little cage."

—John Steinbeck *East of Eden*

People who meet me and learn that I am a psychiatrist often wonder aloud about the relationship between psychiatry and other mental health professions, like psychology. Frequently, they stop themselves midsentence, content they have recalled the essential difference: "You're the ones who can use medicines, right?" they ask.

The stock response to that question is *yes*. We are, of course, physicians empowered to prescribe medication. But that quick answer doesn't really begin to explain the special ways we think about mental illnesses and those who suffer with them.

The foundation of our perspective is built long before we treat our first patients. As first- and second-year medical students, we immerse ourselves in sciences such as biochemistry, physiology, neuroscience,

11

anatomy and pathology. We begin to learn the exquisite balance between structure and function in all organs of the human body.

We come to understand, for example, not simply that excessive dietary fat can lead to heart disease, but how the fat is broken down chemically by the stomach, pancreas and intestine, how it is deposited in atherosclerotic plaques that block arteries, and the dynamics by which blood flow can itself contribute to the developing obstruction. We study slides that show us the microscopic structure of blood vessels choked by fatty deposits. We cut open the large arteries of our cadavers and find the blockages for ourselves.

We learn that the metabolism of sugar and fat are linked and that other illnesses, like diabetes, can accelerate the atherosclerotic process. Looking at dozens of diseases, we continually find abnormalities in one organ disturbing the precarious equilibriums of others. We gain a healthy respect for the intricacy of the body systems we are entrusted to care for.

We become biological skeptics, doubters not only of simple answers, but of simple questions. Early on, our professors dissuade us from any embarrassment that might once have come from saying, "I don't know." In the spirit of discovery, we second- and third-guess each other and ourselves.

We begin to understand that our own medical treatments, aimed at single abnormalities, can have domino side effects elsewhere in the body. Some drugs used to lower fats in the bloodstream, for example, can cause kidney dysfunction and skin problems. They may even be associated with an increased risk of cancer.

And this is just the beginning. We learn that a person's habits, including smoking, alcohol consumption and level of physical activity, can hasten or delay cardiac disease. We debate how important these variables are compared with the individual's genetic makeup. Can people, we wonder aloud, escape family histories rife with heart attack by living differently?

Such questions, we are told, must be answered scientifically. We cannot expect an impression of a problem, or even long experience with it, to yield reliable solutions. Clinical lore is only the seed of discovery. Theories about smoking and heart disease, for example, must be tested in scientific investigations in which hundreds or thousands of patients are objectively studied. The beliefs of the investigators can so subtly and significantly influence the results that when a drug is under study, it will often be given to only half the patients enrolled, and the researchers will learn which half only after all the resulting effects have been catalogued and analyzed.

We dissect cadavers systematically, obsessively tracing the routes of nerves and blood vessels, as if to prove the existence of the systems we have studied. We find physical evidence of illness—hearts overgrown with the effort of pumping against blocked arteries, limbs paralyzed in life and shriveled from disuse, cancers of every variety.

We try to blunt the transition from books to flesh by telling morbid jokes about the human body that, to an outsider, would seem the height of callousness. We capriciously name our cadavers. We laugh nervously at warnings in the dissection manual that we guard our eyes against the fragments of bone loosed by our saws.

Our very attempts to distance ourselves, however, confirm that the pathology has been humanized. We begin to find evidence of lives lived—broken and healed bones, scars, lungs turned black from deep breaths of smoke. We call home and urge parents to stop smoking. It may be no accident that we end our dissections with the head and neck, beginning to look death in the face.

But it is on the wards that the face of mortality has a voice and a family and feels pain and has unrealized dreams.

It was during medical school at Johns Hopkins that a man with lung cancer, dying on a respirator, scrawled out a note urging me to take a break from caring for him and get myself something to eat. It was there that a black man who had worked as a janitor and was wasting away from alcoholism and uncontrolled diabetes sparkled as he told me of the six children he had sent through college. On these same wards, a mother whose son was suffering his fourth life-threatening infection from AIDS asked me how many times she would have to die with him.

I saw Dr. Frank Oski, chairman of pediatrics, cry as he warned our class never to take away hope from terminally ill children.

There are many questions, we learn, that looking under a microscope did not prepare us for. We struggle to understand why the same pathology that causes some people great preoccupation and constant pain, seems less ravaging in those who speak of *refusing* to give up. We wonder why one person might wait ten years to seek medical attention for a growing skin cancer, while another returns to the clinic time and time again, petrified over harmless blemishes. We find, ultimately, that the biochemical reactions and anatomic structures we memorized in class were just the beginning of an understanding of human illness.

Those of us who choose to study psychiatry tend to be fascinated, rather than irritated, by such intangibles. We enter specialty training knowing that ours will be a field steeped in the ambiguity that comes from profound questions about what makes human beings think, feel and act. Are we simply intricate circuitry that sometimes fails? Will the evolution of medical technology allow us to visualize and fix the broken parts? Or must we be content that the sum of a human being will always be immeasurably greater than the collection of its parts? Could it be that we can connect with, but never dissect, the soul? And would that be a gain or a loss?

Even before my residency training in psychiatry, then, some of the groundwork for my treatment of Oliver had been laid. I was able to conceive of a connection between his psychotic thinking and neuro-chemical abnormalities in his brain—chaos in the system of chemical messengers carrying information from one nerve cell to another. I knew that overactivity of dopamine might be at fault and that antipsychotic medication could help bring that system back toward equilibrium.

I also knew that brain chemistry might simply have been the last domino to fall. Disorder in one body system can disrupt another. Diseases affecting the thyroid gland or adrenal gland, for example, can grossly change a person's behavior and thought process. So can a stroke or physical trauma to the brain. A complete medical and psychiatric history would be essential to Oliver's care.

I would have to know his personal habits. Illicit drug abuse (and certain prescription medications) can cause temporary or lasting psychosis. Conversely, withdrawal from alcohol can cause transient psychotic thinking.

Because some mental illnesses—such as schizophrenia and depression—run in families, I would need to know whether his relatives had ever suffered from any.

But all this would only be a beginning. There were other, less concrete, questions to be answered. Why now had Oliver's life taken a turn into such dramatic illness? Were there unresolved issues in his marriage that had complicated the grieving process over his wife's death? What was the nature of his relationship with his daughter? Was he made vulnerable by an emotional Achilles' heel from childhood traumas? Why did his psychosis take the form of an imposter in his midst, rather than a monstrous voice or vision? Accepting that his brain was somehow sick, how was his mind involved in his illness?

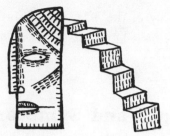

3

The Art of Psychiatric Diagnosis

What can we expect from this path? We can expect the results that Osler promised and delivered to medicine itself: an understanding of the differences among the patients we see and eventually an appreciation of the varieties of etiology and mechanism found in different psychiatric disorders.

—Paul R. McHugh, M.D., Chief of Psychiatry,
Johns Hopkins University School of Medicine

This may be the most difficult chapter in this book to read. It is the hardest for me to write. It is about organization and labeling—about how psychiatry uses the similarities between patients to predict how they will respond to certain kinds of treatments, including medications. As such, it carries with it the same potential for emotional detachment as writing about surgery. The inherent peril is that we could come to focus on naming illnesses at the expense of understanding the individuals they afflict.

If you share my hunger for interpersonal poetry in the pages that follow, this chapter will have achieved one of its goals. You will already live in the household of psychiatry's uneasy marriage to medical science. For although no two individuals have the same life story—and no one's pain can be completely described by anyone else's—our diagnostic vocabulary consists only of the 300 or so disorders catalogued in the American Psychiatric Association's *Diagnostic and Statistical Manual of Mental Disorders* (DSM).

Signs and Symptoms

Unlike most medical illnesses, patients with psychiatric conditions may have no demonstrable bodily abnormality in common. We often can't point to a damaged organ or a hormone deficiency as proof that a particular illness is present. We assign patients a diagnosis because of consistencies among them in the way they act and the way they feel. But we know that a 300-word language cannot comfortably encompass their suffering. This inherent limitation of our diagnostic manual partly accounts for the fact that many psychiatrists remain uncomfortable that the DSM classifications are overzealous—artificially grouping patients together.

As constraining as it can be, however, our diagnostic vocabulary has real power to help people. It has been developed by carefully examining countless patients in an effort to document recurring patterns of signs (characteristics a physician observes) and symptoms (complaints a patient reports). Only once these common *syndromes* are identified can the biochemical, anatomic and even psychological mechanisms underlying them be effectively studied. Treatments can be tailored to interfere with the specific gears of illness that are at work in each condition.

We have learned, for example, that major depression consists of more than low mood.[†] We now ask patients whether they are experiencing other known symptoms, such as fatigue, feelings of worthlessness, decreased ability to concentrate and thoughts of death or suicide. We expect that appetite may be affected, with resulting weight loss or, less commonly, weight gain. We pay attention to how much the patient moves, because we know that excessive or greatly diminished activity is frequently present.

[†]The complete DSM-III-R diagnostic criteria for a major depressive episode and major depression may be found in Appendix A.

We also know that depression often occurs as part of a cycling mood condition marked by both highs and lows (bipolar disorder). The questions we ask of a depressed patient, therefore, will include whether he or she has ever experienced the euphoria, grandiosity, decreased need for sleep, risk-taking behavior and rapid speech typical of mania.[†]

Distinguishing between the diagnoses (the process of *differential diagnosis*) is critical. Antidepressant medication may suffice for those patients with uncomplicated major depression, but a different mood stabilizer, such as lithium, may be indicated for those who cycle from high to low. Moreover, using certain antidepressants in susceptible patients can actually bring about a manic episode.

One tool psychiatrists use to elicit and organize signs and symptoms is the *mental status examination*. As we speak with a patient, we are attentive, first of all, to his or her **appearance.** Does the patient seem comfortable or agitated? Is he or she well groomed or disheveled? Are there signs suggesting that drug or alcohol use is involved?

The patient's appearance alone may provide invaluable information about his or her current symptoms and past history. We may notice that the patient's eyes dart here and there, as if tracking an illusory voice or vision. He or she may look fearful when there is no apparent threat. Signs of *tardive dyskinesia*, an occasionally debilitating movement disorder that sometimes follows the prolonged use of antipsychotic medications, may be evident.

In Oliver's case, his dark lenses, together with the fact that he moved his seat as far from mine as possible, made me wonder if he was paranoid. The neatness of his clothing told me that he had not completely lost the ability to concentrate and attend to his hygiene (as some very depressed or psychotic patients do). His overalls and bright red bandana were colorful, but not as provocative as the clothing chosen by some manic patients. He had no apparent abnormalities of movement—not the tremor that can come with taking too much lithium, not the restlessness that is a common side effect of antipsychotic medication, not

---

[†]The complete DSM-III-R diagnostic criteria for mania may be found in Appendix B.

the lack of movement that might result from depression, schizophrenia or brain injury.

By contrast, I have met patients in the emergency room who, although they had the facial movements typical of tardive dyskinesia, assured me they had never before seen a psychiatrist. Most often, further knowledge of their histories (from families or physicians or from old medical records) revealed extensive psychiatric illness.

As psychiatrists watch, we listen, not only for the thematic content of the patient's **speech,** but also for its rate, tone and idiosyncrasies. Manic patients tend to speak too quickly (called *pressured* speech). Depressed or schizophrenic patients may speak little or not at all (*poverty of speech* or *mutism*). Those patients who have neurological impairment, such as from repeated small strokes, may have difficulty finding words or enunciating. Patients suffering from hallucinations sometimes respond verbally to voices only they can hear or visions only they can see. Those with disordered thinking may invent words with special meaning (*neologisms*) or repeat everything said to them (*echolalia*).

Oliver's speech was normal. I have treated other patients, however, whose speech patterns were like calling cards for their disorders. I introduced myself to one manic patient, for example, who immediately expressed his hope that I would be someone he might "pray with and stay with." He then rushed through a staccato series of loosely connected rhymes.

While it is tempting to think of the mental status examination as psychiatry's equivalent of a physical examination, this is not like listening to the heart for a murmur. When psychiatric illness is audible, we understand that we must go beyond documenting the sounds of suffering. We are always attempting to connect emotionally with the *person* suffering. We are like cardiologists open to the idea that our stethoscopes might reveal arrhythmias to one ear and broken hearts to the other.

In an attempt to gauge the likelihood of an affective disorder being present, we ask the patient to rate his or her **mood.** Sometimes we suggest that the patient use a 10-point scale, with 1 being the worst mood he or she has ever experienced and 10 being the best.

The portrait of the patient becomes more complete as we ponder his or her **affect**—the observable manifestations of emotion. Is the patient, for example, displaying a full range of facial expression, or does he or she look consistently despondent (depressed affect) or emotionless (blunted affect)? Is he or she tearful? Is the patient's emotional expression consistent with mood (mood-congruent affect), or are the two seemingly disconnected (as when a patient reports feeling depressed, but laughs consistently)? Does the patient's affect seem to reflect the topic being discussed, or is there emotional detachment from what seem to be evocative subjects?

My initial interview with Oliver made me focus on the possibility of a mood disorder because he reported feeling irritable and was emotionally labile, swinging easily from tears to anger.

I didn't run through the mental status examination as if it were a checklist. A physical examination proceeds in regimented fashion from head and neck, to heart and lungs, to arms and legs. The mental status examination takes shape as the patient tells his or her story. The psychiatrist learns the most by actively listening. Certain facts must eventually be recorded, but the art of the interview is to gather these as gifts of insight offered by the patient, rather than as information methodically collected by the clinician. The beauty of the initial psychiatric assessment is in the fluidity with which a skilled clinician and a troubled patient together sketch the parameters of the problems at hand.

These are drawn, in part, by the patient's **thought content** and **thought process**—roughly translated, the substance and organization of the ideas occupying him or her. Psychiatrists are initially interested in whether a patient is suicidal, homicidal or paranoid and whether thoughts come in organized fashion or not. Some patients, for example, complain that thoughts are rushing too quickly through their minds (*flight of ideas*, consistent with mania). Others relate thoughts that seem to have little connection to one another (*loosening of associations*, typical of psychotic thinking).

Like Oliver, patients may suffer from tenaciously held, false beliefs called *delusions*. A delusion central to Oliver's suffering, of course, was his paranoid conviction that his daughter had been kidnapped and replaced by a double. His belief that he had been raised by celebrities was a *delusion of grandeur*.

I was careful to find out that Oliver was neither suicidal nor homicidal, because one of my central responsibilities to him was ensuring that he was not an immediate risk to himself or others.

The unfolding of a patient's thought content often takes place over several sessions, making differential diagnosis a gradual process. The patient may reveal a troubling delusion, for example, only after he or she is convinced that the therapist is trustworthy.

Thought content can also change abruptly. A patient may be paranoid while under the influence of cocaine, but perfectly rational hours later. He or she may threaten suicide in the emergency room, but feel safe enough once on an inpatient ward to disavow any harmful intent.

The same is true of **perceptions.** Patients may freely share that they are troubled by hallucinations (such as hearing voices or seeing visions) or may deny these experiences even when they are terrified by them. Moreover, hallucinations may herald a major mental illness or be limited to periods preceding seizures or to episodes of drug use or drug withdrawal.

As is the case in listening to the patient's speech, we are not satisfied simply to note that a patient hears voices. We gain valuable insight into that person's suffering from how the voices sound and what they say. Are the voices recognizable? Are they threatening? Do they, as is typical in some forms of depression, demean the patient? Do they demand that an act of violence be committed?

The mental status examination also includes questions designed to assess a patient's **cognitive abilities,** including memory, concentration and awareness of time and place—all of which can change dramatically from day to day.

Any single mental status examination is, after all, only the equivalent of one frame in a motion picture. To more fully understand the patient's distress and predict how it might evolve in the future, we rely heavily on lessons from the past.

Past Psychiatric History

Illnesses, like people, have histories. Some are born, grow strong, are beaten back and lay quiet between periods of terrible activity. Some rage for a time, only to be vanquished entirely. Others never surrender the ground they gain. While psychiatrists must be students of the life stories of our patients, performing differential diagnosis also requires focusing on the life histories of the disorders that visit them.

We know, for example, that depression and mania tend to be *episodic*—they come and go. Similarly, alcohol dependence may remit for a time, only to resurface months, years or even decades later. Schizophrenia, on the other hand, is a constant, chronic illness that generally takes an increasing toll on the social and occupational functioning of its victims.

Disorders are also typically born at different times in their victims' lives. Depression can occur throughout life—in children or the elderly. Schizophrenia rarely begins before age ten or after age forty. Anorexia nervosa is most common in teenagers.

Symptoms of constricted affect, social withdrawal and paranoia that begin at age fifty, for example, are more likely due to major depression than to schizophrenia, especially if the symptoms are recurring after a period of good health and function.

Oliver denied any psychiatric symptoms before age thirty-nine, when he lost his wife. This, together with the fact that he had abruptly (rather than gradually) declined from a high level of functioning, made me think of schizophrenia as an unlikely culprit.

Sometimes we learn about one disorder by inquiring about the company it has kept with others. Alcohol, which ultimately makes matters worse, can provide temporary relief from unstable mood, anxiety or insomnia. Some patients find it quiets the distressing voices they hear. The past psychiatric history of an alcoholic patient, therefore, might lead us to suspect that the addiction began as a misguided attempt to relieve symptoms of panic disorder, posttraumatic stress disorder or a mood disorder.

The history of a psychiatric disorder is further revealed through its relationship with the health care delivery system. The need for repeated or very lengthy hospitalizations generally indicates that symptoms were too serious to manage in an outpatient setting. Unsuccessful trials of many different medications suggest that side effects may have been severe, or that symptoms were especially resistant to treatment.

There were other lessons I gathered from Oliver's psychiatric history. He had never been assaultive, never attempted suicide and never been hospitalized against his will. These facts testified to a history of self-control that gave me some confidence he could remain safely in the community.

I know that none of the reasoning I have described thus far speaks to Oliver's singular life experiences or to the dramatic themes of abandonment and isolation which an empathic ear cannot miss hearing in his symptoms. The initial attempt to catalogue a patient's past psychiatric history is necessarily organizational and scientific, rather than thematic.

Family Psychiatric and Medical Histories

Some psychiatric and medical illnesses can touch multiple family members and span generations. Psychiatrists, therefore, elicit detailed family trees to assess whether a patient might be at increased risk for a given condition, perhaps based on a genetic predisposition. This is particularly helpful as we attempt to settle on the correct diagnosis in an individual who suffers symptoms that may be caused by one of several disorders.

The fact that Oliver's father seemed to have suffered episodes of depression and mania reinforced my belief that Oliver's delusional thinking was part of a protracted mood disorder. I wondered whether his mother's alcoholism meant that she, too, had been struggling with mood swings.

Although controversial, a genetic tendency toward suicide has even been theorized. Had Oliver's father or mother taken his or her own life, I would have been especially concerned about Oliver's personal safety.

The family psychiatric history can be helpful in selecting among available treatments, as well. In psychoses that are resistant to medication, for example, a good response in one ill family member is a clue that the same medicine may work in another family member.

Because medical conditions can cause psychiatric illness (as discussed later in this chapter), the medical histories of family members are also important data in a patient's differential diagnosis. Diabetes, for example, can result in extreme fatigue, lethargy and clouded thinking. These symptoms, in a patient whose parents are diabetic, would make a psychiatrist particularly suspicious that abnormal sugar metabolism might be to blame.

Again, although differential diagnosis relies heavily on scientific reasoning, this does not change the fact that one person's illness can reverberate emotionally in others. Aside from potential genetic predispositions, the family history can illuminate a patient's early life experiences. If, as in Oliver's case, substance abuse or multiple hospitalizations or chronic medical illness made a parent emotionally unavailable, we might well find evidence of that early trauma in the patient's adult relationships.

Alcohol and Illicit Drug History

The immediate and lasting impact of alcohol and other drugs on mental health is so powerful that a history of abuse or dependence can nearly paralyze the process of psychiatric diagnosis. The paranoia sparked by cocaine, the immediate hallucinations and "flashbacks" caused by LSD, and the altered thinking linked to alcoholism can mimic other serious psychiatric illnesses.

For this reason, obtaining a detailed history of alcohol and illicit drug use is essential in treating patients. A snapshot view of a cocaine user who has stopped taking the drug, for example, can look just like major depression, with low mood and irritability persisting for months.

Even more complicated, alcohol and illicit drugs often gain a foothold in emotional ground made ready by another psychiatric disorder. The cocaine user who stops and falls victim to depressive symptoms may be experiencing simple withdrawal, but might also be experiencing the reemergence of a chronic depressive state he or she attempted to relieve with the drug.

Our task is often to determine whether a patient's signs and symptoms will resolve with abstinence or whether they will persist, either because of lasting damage from drugs or because of another underlying psychiatric condition. Differential diagnosis in those patients impaired by alcohol or illicit drugs, therefore, is often a lengthy process, with final diagnosis deferred until the patient is alcohol or drug free.

Medical History

Many of us who ultimately choose to practice psychiatry worry over leaving our white coats behind, letting our hard-won knowledge of physical diseases fade away. In fact, the fear is unwarranted. A patient's mental status and physical condition are often so closely linked that the art of psychiatric diagnosis depends on a complete working knowledge of the human body.

The intertwined roots of psychiatric and medical illness are most apparent when a patient suffers psychiatric symptoms due to an underlying bodily abnormality. Lessons from medical school about disorder in one body organ visiting chaos upon another become animate as we meet patients in whom, for example, overproduction of a hormone is causing hallucinations, or impaired breathing is causing marked confusion. Depressed mood and decreased energy may reflect an underlying cancer. Extreme anxiety can result from cardiac abnormalities such as mitral valve prolapse.

Medications that are used to treat physical illness can also cause psychiatric symptoms. Curing a patient who suffers with sadness, tearfulness, impotence and fatigue can sometimes be as easy as changing the medicine he or she takes for high blood pressure.

For these and other reasons, the key to a proper diagnosis of emotional suffering is often found in the patient's medical, rather than psychiatric, history.

In Oliver's case, knowing that Capgras' syndrome has been associated with head trauma, I was particularly interested in whether he had ever hurt his head badly or suffered seizures. I was also careful to look for ongoing signs of brain injury. An abnormal gait, for example, would have made me more suspicious that Oliver might be showing signs of a brain tumor or a stroke.

The connections between psychiatric and medical illness run both ways. Physical signs and symptoms are sometimes caused by an underlying psychiatric condition. These can range from vague aches and pains to blindness. I have met patients in whom terrible chest pain (requiring monitoring in the intensive care unit) responded completely to antianxiety medication, and others in whom depression manifested itself as partial paralysis.

Medical history can also be linked more subtly with psychiatric symptoms. Illnesses have meaning to patients. Seemingly minor physical conditions can be psychologically devastating. Whereas hernia surgery, for example, may be routine for one man, another may become depressed, viewing the breach in his muscles as the beginning of physical infirmity and old age. One patient may seem to take heart disease in stride, whereas another, whose mother or father died young from a heart attack, may become fearful of any physical exertion and withdraw from others.

Sandy, a middle-aged woman admitted to the hospital with major depression, had been working as a meat cutter until she suffered a back injury. The grocery store had reassigned her to a position as an assistant manager, because strenuous physical labor would no longer be possible. "I was as strong as any man there," she said. "And now I can't even pull my own weight."

"You don't feel you do a good job as a manager?" I asked.

"That's a joke, not a job," she said. "Who calls walking around the aisles real work?"

It was easier to understand how deeply affected Sandy was by her injury once she explained more about her father, a carpenter who often worked sixteen-hour days.

"My father only spent time with my brothers," she said, "until it turned out that I was better helping out with his work than they were. I could square beams better. I could drive nails better. I did it all."

Sandy's physical injury, laced as it was with early feelings about the essential role of physical strength in winning her father's affection, was central to understanding her psychiatric illness.

Her suffering is also key to understanding the art of psychiatric assessment, diagnosis and treatment. For even though she did suffer from depression, even though that illness was indeed related to a physical injury, the language of science cannot explain the connection. The diagnostic labels of major depression and ruptured intervertebral disk— while helpful in describing her condition—do not adequately capture her experience.

Psychiatrists must consistently listen to patients in a variety of ways. We need to listen for the signs and symptoms that distinguish one psychiatric diagnosis from another. We need to listen for medical information that might disclose a bodily abnormality underlying those signs and symptoms. And, always, we need to listen for the meaning, the music, that can turn seemingly inert facts into a rich and uniquely human story.

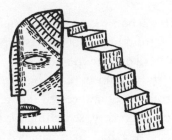

4

The Woman With Burning Feet

Physical pain is a common language. Whatever our backgrounds, beliefs and values, a painful grimace requires no translation. It speaks directly to the empathic core in each of us. We all understand, perhaps from the moment we are born, what it means to hurt.

It should be no surprise, then, that pain can be the calling card for many forms of psychiatric distress. When we do not, or cannot, put our anguish into words, the brain seems capable of independently raising this universal red flag.

Maria, who visited me on the advice of her internist, was no complainer. She was seventy-seven years old and had worked as a seamstress, without missing a single day, for over forty of those years. She had raised a family, tolerated a divorce and managed living alone for a decade. She had survived severe bouts of pneumonia and a heart attack. Her body was stout in a way that suggested solidity, rather than indulgence.

As if to say that words would indeed fail her, Maria took off her ankle boots and knee highs just moments after she sat down in my office. She drew in a deep breath and began rubbing her feet. Her eyes welled up.

Portions of this chapter were first published in *The Washington Post*.

I knew from a letter I had received from her internist that Maria's feet burned ceaselessly, from her ankles to the tips of her toes. A team of doctors, including a vascular surgeon and a neurologist, had searched for a bodily abnormality that could explain her suffering. They had measured the blood flow to her feet and tested the nerves and muscles. They had analyzed her blood chemistry, searching for the uric acid of gout or the sugar of diabetes. They had even imaged the base of her spine, where nerves serving the feet originate, to make sure no tumor or deformity of bone was interfering with them. They could find no explanation.

"You're in terrible pain," I observed.

Maria gestured with upturned palms toward her feet. "Look for yourself," she said. "Look how red they are. They burn like fire. They send me to a psychiatrist. Who *wouldn't* be depressed with feet like these?" She shook her head.

I wanted Maria to know that I didn't assume her problem was psychiatric; often physical causes of pain do go undetected for long periods of time. I also wanted her to know that nothing about her feet was repulsive *to me*. "May I look at them?" I asked.

She nodded hesitantly. I kneeled down and held both of her feet in my hands. She took another deep breath.

"Am I hurting you?" I asked.

"They hurt all the time."

I felt the strong pulses at her ankles. I asked her to close her eyes and raise a hand when I touched her toes. Her perfect performance showed she could sense light touch.

"It's not just in my head," she said once I had sat down again.

"I believe you have pain," I said. She seemed to relax a bit. "I wonder how this pain has affected your life."

"Ruined me," she said. "I can't sleep. I wake up four, five in the morning. I don't go out for walks anymore. I don't feel so much like eating. Two months already, and no doctor can tell me what's wrong. They do tests and more tests."

"Has your ability to concentrate been affected?"

"I can't read the newspaper, even," she said, shaking her head, again.

The fact that Maria's pain was accompanied by low mood, together with symptoms of early morning awakening, loss of appetite, decreased concentration and decreased activity, made me consider whether a depression was to blame. Were pain her only symptom, I would have suspected the more circumscribed condition called *somatoform pain disorder*.[†]

Although she denied past depressive episodes (and had no family history of mood disorders), depression is more common in the elderly and in those who feel isolated. The highly treatable memory deficits and confusion typical of depression, in fact, are often tragically mistaken for irreversible Alzheimer's disease.

It is also not unusual for physical symptoms to be among the most prominent complaints of those suffering from major depression. No one is certain why this should be. It may be that the same abnormalities of chemical messengers in the brain that are responsible for low mood also lower the body's pain threshold. It might be that early learning has integrated into our unconscious the idea that only physical distress will reliably elicit care from others. Perhaps the aches and pains associated with depression are some virulent cousin of the stomachaches that sweep children on the first day of school.

"This pain is affecting more than your feet," I said. "If we could meet weekly, and I could learn more about you, I think we might start to control some of the ways it has changed your life."

Maria agreed. She slowly laced on her black leather boots. As she walked out of the clinic, I noticed that she winced with each step.

She telephoned my office a few days later to tell me that the pain was no worse, but no better. She still wasn't sleeping or eating well. I listened a few minutes, encouraged that we had made an attachment. Before saying good-bye, I started to reassure her that we would have more time to talk when she came for her second appointment.

"So how is your day?" she interrupted.

"Things are fine here," I said.

"O.K., then, I'll be by to see you soon."

Maria's tone, increasingly from the beginning of our conversation to the end, was warm and familiar. She had led with an update on her

---

[†]The complete diagnostic criteria for somatoform pain disorder may be found in Appendix C.

condition, but I also sensed her need to take care of *me*. Before I could reassure her by confirming our second appointment, in fact, she had interrupted with her own promise to visit.

Who was I to this woman, I wondered? I was, of course, her doctor, on the surface of it. But under cover of our respective roles as physician and patient, I felt she was treating me more like a son or, perhaps, a grandson. Our conversation left me wanting to assert my adulthood and professionalism. To me, this internal observation was data as essential as the results of studies on her nerves and muscles. Something intimately mixed up with the pain that had brought her to my office was alive in the nurturing manner with which she inquired after my day.

At the start of our second meeting, Maria went through the same ritual that had marked our first. She unlaced her black boots, removed her hosiery and began to rub her feet. "Look at them," she said, motioning with both hands. "Red like flames. You can examine them, if you want."

I read her invitation both as a symbol of trust and a test of faith. At the same time as acknowledging that I might be helpful to her, she was reminding me that her problem, presumably manifest on physical examination, was *real*, not *in her head*. Examining her feet might be the admission ticket I needed in order to gain access to her life.

I crouched down and held her feet, again. Then I performed the simple tests I had done the week before.

"You're still in pain," I said, taking my seat.

"Pain like you wouldn't believe." She began to cry.

I sat a full minute with her as she wept.

She wiped her eyes. "I have no right to be so unhappy," she said, looking down at her feet. "I've had a full life."

"What have you most enjoyed?"

"My family," she said, and the tears threatened to start, again.

"Is the family well?"

"Thank God. I even got a letter from my grandson that he's fine. You know something . . ." She stared at me. "He looks a little like you." She smiled. "Now, there's a boy. Smarter than his teachers, they said when he was in high school. He likes those computers."

"Is he away at college now?" I asked.

"He's in Saudi Arabia. In the army," she said.

I looked at her for several seconds without saying a word. I nodded slowly. When I did speak I did so quietly, as if I might scare off the poetry I suspected was just around the corner. "How long has he been there?"

"Oh, about two months, I guess."

The coincidence in time of Maria's pain and her grandson's departure was irresistible. I nodded, again. I felt a mixture of wonder, excitement, embarrassment and fear. Could it be that Maria was empathically *with* her grandson in the desert? Had her love for him transcended the usual boundaries of person, place and time?

"What does your grandson say it's like in Saudi Arabia?" I asked cautiously.

"It's a desert," she said. She shrugged and glanced at her feet. "Hot sand everywhere."

I was silent again. My eyes moved to her feet, as if her feet might, under the pressure of direct inquiry, confess their intrigue. "Does your grandson's being in the desert have anything to do with your feet?" I asked.

She looked back at them. For a moment, we were both gazing down. "I don't see how it could," she said, breaking the spell. The connection seemed to disturb her. "No. One thing has nothing to do with the other. It couldn't be."

Knowing how important it had been to Maria for me to conceive of her pain as a bodily abnormality, I didn't want to force its symbolism on her. "It seemed a striking coincidence is all," I said dismissively. "What with your feet burning and your grandson at war in the desert . . . It was just a thought."

She seemed to need to reinforce the physical signs and dispel their possible emotional meaning. She grimaced and began rubbing her feet. "It's like they're buried in hot coals," she said. "They're burning up." She began to cry. "Can't you give me anything for the pain?"

I had already considered prescribing a tricyclic antidepressant for Maria. In moderate dosages, such medications are known not only to treat symptoms of depression but also to relieve some kinds of chronic pain. Although their mechanism of action is not entirely understood, we do know that tricyclics enhance the action of the brain chemical messengers norepinephrine and serotonin.

In offering medication to her, I knew that manipulating Maria's serotonin and norepinephrine might or might not be responsible for any future improvement. Even if her pain and other symptoms were reduced over the coming weeks, it would be impossible to decipher, with absolute confidence, precisely why. After all, Maria and I had already established a relationship that might be reassuring to her. She had commented that I even *looked* like her grandson. We had also uncovered (although she initially rejected it) the apparent meaning of her pain, a discovery from which she might slowly take comfort. And the very act of my prescribing medicine (thus taking Maria's pain seriously) might in and of itself be some relief to her.

Two days later, Maria phoned, again. "I'm not sure this medicine is working," she said. "I can't tell if the pain is any better."

Her ambivalence about the continued severity of her pain made me hopeful. "It may take several days or even a few weeks for you to feel better," I reassured her. "But I think the medicine will help."

"I'll be seeing you on Friday?" she asked.

"Yes. I'll certainly see you Friday."

"You have a good week, then," she said.

When we met, Maria did not repeat her ritual of removing her boots and asking me to examine her feet. Instead, she immediately dug into her handbag and found two newspaper clippings, which she unfolded and placed on my desk. "That's my grandson," she said, pointing to a photograph in the center of one of the articles. "That's when he got his computer science award in high school. He's a scientist, like you. And that one there," she pointed to the second article, "is when he made the high honor roll."

"A very smart boy," I observed.

"Smarter than his teachers, is what they all said. Always with a book, my grandson. He loves to read. Some of the time I can't even follow what he says, but he's got a heart of gold, let me tell you . . ."

Maria and I spoke about her grandson for most of the hour. Not until the end of the session did I address her pain. "Have your feet improved?" I asked, pointing at them.

She seemed surprised that her feet should still be the topic of our discussion. She looked down at them. "Much better," she said. "I can finally sleep and I'm walking again. That pill you gave me is a wonder drug."

"It's good medicine," I said.

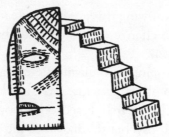

5

Oliver, Maria and Psychiatry's
Diagnostic and Statistical Manual

The whole field seemed like a highway filled with angry drivers curs-
ing each other and telling each other they didn't know how to drive
when the real trouble was the highway itself. The highway had been
laid down as the scientific objective study of man in a manner that
paralleled the physical sciences. . . . Objects of scientific study are supposed to hold still. They're supposed to follow the laws of cause and
effect in such a way that a given cause will always have a given effect,
over and over again. Man doesn't do this. Not even savages.

—Robert M. Pirsig *Lila*

Oliver and Maria both suffer from disorders described in psychiatry's
official diagnostic manual, the *Diagnostic and Statistical Manual of
Mental Disorders*, Third Edition, Revised (DSM-III-R). In giving them
diagnoses, their signs and symptoms—whether reflecting abnormalities
of mood, thought or perception—are sorted through the field's cumula-
tive experience with patients. Oliver's signs and symptoms are most
similar to those observed in, and reported by, manic patients. Maria's fit

well with depression. Knowing this predicts a great deal about how their conditions are likely to change over time, and about which treatments have proven most helpful.

Yet this kind of grouping into diagnostic categories does not tell us other vital information about patients. First, unlike a medical diagnosis such as diabetes, which is partly based on abnormal levels of glucose measured in the blood, psychiatric diagnoses are not based on organic and measurable underlying pathology. They don't offer the same confidence that physiological gears need only be set right for health to be restored. Moreover, while the categories attempt to describe how one disorder differs in presentation from another, they don't speak at all to the crucial psychological differences between patients with the *same* disorder. This is why reading the DSM-III-R descriptions of mania and depression feels so different (and, in some ways, so much less satisfying) than reading the case histories of Oliver and Maria. The former describe syndromes; the latter describe people.

It is also why history gathering in psychiatry is so complex. On the one hand, medical school teaches us to be attentive to cataloguing the signs and symptoms with which a patient presents. On the other hand, we know that every patient's suffering is a story, not just a list of complaints. To think we can encompass the range of that suffering using a 300-word diagnostic vocabulary is naive and misleading.

These critical issues have split psychiatry along competing intellectual axes almost from its inception. Sigmund Freud himself embodied the struggle. He began his *Project for a Scientific Psychology* in 1895, convinced that mental life could be explained in terms of the properties of single brain cells exchanging quantities of energy between one another. He wrote that his intention was to "furnish a psychology that shall be a natural science: that is, to represent psychical processes as quantitatively determinate states . . ."

Freud was, after all, a gifted clinician and researcher who shared with today's physicians extensive experience with, and great respect for, the anatomic and physiologic underpinnings of illness. Like us, he dissected a cadaver, studied slides of damaged tissues, and examined patients with debilitating medical and neurological disorders. Like us, he witnessed the power of cures directed at the bodily gears of disease. Yet, within a few years of starting his quest for a scientific psychology, he realized that the biochemical, physiologic and anatomic information at hand failed to explain the mental phenomena he was observing in patients.

Faced with this intellectual gulf, Freud made a critical decision: He introduced into his system the conceptual bridge of an "ego," a kind of all-knowing managing partner in each of us that buries painful early experiences. These early traumas, often sexual in nature, do not sit calmly underground. They take root and grow back to the surface, no longer recognizable for what they were, but disguised as symptoms like paralysis and psychosis. Only if patients can be helped to recall the early traumas and to release the emotional energy connected with them, Freud maintained, will the symptoms disappear.

Freud knew that the ego would never be dissected from a cadaver or seen under a microscope. It wasn't borne of objective science. The idea constitutes an intuitive and useful parable about the causes of psychiatric illness, a kind of universal story line to begin deciphering a myriad of personal dramas. Near the end of his life, Freud wrote the following:

> We know two kinds of things about what we call our psyche (or mental life): firstly, its bodily organ and scene of action, the brain (or nervous system) and, on the other hand, our acts of consciousness, which are immediate data and cannot be further explained by any sort of description. Everything that lies between is unknown to us, and the data do not include any direct relation between these two terminal points of our knowledge. If it existed, it would at the most afford an exact localization of the processes of consciousness and would give us no help towards understanding them.

Psychiatrists today sometimes forget that our field has always drawn its strength from integrating these disparate medical model and life story approaches to healing emotional distress and mental disorders. We have managed to sustain what other medical specialties only now aspire to—a promising partnership of biological and psychological understandings. As the case of Samuel will illustrate, these two, far from being natural enemies, turn out to be chambers of one heart.

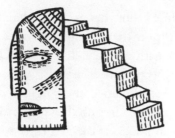

6

The Flood

"See?" Samuel said, staring at his right hand. "It's already starting to fall. We're in for it. Horrible things are going to happen."

Samuel's right arm, bent vertically at the elbow, was resting on his thigh as he sat hunched at the side of his hospital bed. The hand, like some shell-shocked bird, shook slightly with the effort at hovering midair.

"If you let your hand fall something bad will happen?" I asked.

"*Bad?*" he echoed, incredulous. "You'll drown, is all. You and everyone else in this hospital. Maybe in the world. The water will swallow every last one of you." Panic showed in his aging face as the hand wavered slightly. With his left hand, he grabbed his right wrist to keep the odd bird aloft. "I can't keep this up forever," he said apologetically. "I'm sorry, but I may not be able to save you. It's my fault."

Samuel had been admitted to the medical service with a severe intestinal infection. After a few days in the hospital, he became disoriented, mistaking the year for 1979 and the city for Philadelphia. He confided in his primary physician that he feared the staff might be tired of caring for him, or even trying to harm him. At times he heard rain striking the windows (although it wasn't raining) and saw rivulets of water seeping from the walls.

Portions of this chapter were first published in *The Washington Post*.

41

These kinds of confused thoughts and disordered perceptions are typi-cal of *delirium*, a condition that commonly affects patients, especially the elderly, who suffer with medical disorders.[†] Delirious patients tend to have fluctuating levels of consciousness, with clear thinking at one time during the day and somnolence or disorganized thinking at another.

There is always an organic abnormality responsible. Typical causes of delirium include infection, lack of oxygen to the brain, abnormal levels of various ions in the blood, and medication side effects. A patient's altered mental status, in fact, may be the first clue to an emerging medical problem, such as a urinary tract infection.

While we know that delirium is linked to such bodily conditions, we don't know the precise chemical changes in the brain responsible for the disordered thinking. Nor do we understand why one delirious pa-tient might be panicked and paranoid, while another might comment calmly that strange animals are grazing about the room.

Samuel stood up suddenly, careful to keep his arm bent and immo-bile, and inspected the bag of IV fluid suspended above. "No matter what I do, it keeps dripping," he said, sitting down again. He focused intensely on his bent arm. "I don't know how long I can keep you alive. You see I'm trying my hardest. I'm sorry."

"Are you afraid *you'll* die?" I asked.

"I'll be the last to go down," he said, shaking his head. "I don't know why it has to be, but I'll survive every last one of you. I have to watch all of you sink before it's my turn to go." He grabbed his wrist, again. "You can see I'm doing absolutely everything I can."

I knew enough about Samuel's symptoms to know that his treatment would have to include a meticulous search for the organic cause of his altered mental status. His intestinal infection was an obvious possible culprit, but it might be that his breathing or the blood supply to his brain was also compromised. If Samuel had concealed a dependency on alcohol, we might be witnessing a withdrawal phenomenon (*delirium tremens*, or DTs). Perhaps he had a second, as-yet-unknown infection.

[†]The complete DSM-III-R diagnostic criteria for delirium may be found in Appendix D.

One of his multiple medications, possibly the intravenous antibiotic itself, might even be responsible.

An antipsychotic medication is often extremely helpful in blunting the delusions and hallucinations of delirium. I fully expected that using such a medicine, while beginning to treat any underlying bodily abnormality we might discover, would relieve much of Samuel's suffering. But what, I wondered, was I to make of the particular content of his disordered thinking? Why his insistence that he would have to watch the rest of us die? Was it enough to diagnose the phantoms of his mind as delirium, to read them as essential clues to disordered body chemistry, or might his peculiar brand of suffering be understandable on some more basic, human level, as well?

The word *survive* felt like a possible key. Samuel's fear seemed less centered on his own death than on the horror of *outliving* the rest of us, watching us consumed by gathering waters. "Why do you have to be the last to go?" I asked.

"I don't understand it," Samuel said, his eyes filling with tears. "I just know it has to be."

Maybe I was listening to the random discharges of a short-circuited brain, maybe it was folly to try to make any sense of delirium, but *survive* still felt like some sort of higher ground amid the tempest. "Who have you already survived in your life?" I asked.

Samuel stopped fidgeting with the IV tubing running into his right arm. "I've been thinking about him, too," he said.

"Thinking about whom?" I asked.

"Ned. We met in grade school, if you can believe that. Friends for fifty years. I've been thinking how it would have been his birthday yesterday."

"And what took Ned's life?"

"A stroke," Samuel said. "Two strokes. A little one, then the big one that got him."

I nodded. We were silent for several moments. "What damage did the first stroke do?"

Samuel's arm began to fall. He gasped, but caught it. "That was close," he said. "See, it's a matter of time before you go down. I'm sorry. Look at that water on the walls."

"So what damage did the first stroke do?" I asked, again.

"Ruined half his body. Had to use a cane."

"The right side of his body wasn't working," I said.

"How did you know that?" Samuel asked.

"I was just wondering whether losing Ned might be wrapped up somehow with your right arm," I said.

"Possible," Samuel whispered. "I've wondered that."

"Where did Ned recuperate after his first stroke?" I asked.

"Had him over to the house to get his strength up. Looked good, too, until that second one. Big bleed into his brain, that second one."

"Drowned him," I said.

"Might say." Samuel stared at me.

"Did you see it happen?"

"No, I was at work. My daughter was looking after him when it happened."

The thematic structure of Samuel's delirium, even acknowledging its origins in disordered brain metabolism, was captivating. Hundreds of delirious patients might all suffer with paranoia or hallucinations, but Samuel's delirium read like a parable about the chaos that had befallen Ned. Samuel had gone to work, taking his eyes off his friend, and Ned had been engulfed by a wave of blood crashing into his brain. Was it possible that Samuel's delirium created a kind of stage upon which he was replaying the whole tragedy? Was he desperately maintaining a bizarre vigil to save the rest of us?

"You can't prevent a second stroke, no matter how closely you watch someone," I said. "You did everything you could."

"I tried my hardest," Samuel said, his eyes welling up, again. "I don't know what else I could have done."

"There *wasn't* anything else you could have done," I said. "That's the hardest part."

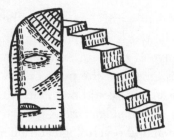

7

A Tapestry of Understandings: The Psychiatric Formulation

It would be a great thing to understand pain in all its meanings.

—Peter Mere Latham *Collected Works* Book I

Each man is ill in his own way.

—Anatole Broyard "Doctor Talk to Me"
New York Times Magazine 1990

Psychiatry may be unique as a medical specialty in the extent to which it has incorporated new knowledge and methods while continuing to value and refine the old. The psychoanalytic theories and life story reasoning of Sigmund Freud, Josef Breuer, Carl Jung and many others have endured, proving useful even in the face of our wonderful new knowledge of neuroanatomy, neurochemistry and genetics. The inherent power of such disparate approaches to understanding and alleviating human suffering has necessarily made of us gatherer-physicians, taking what is most helpful to patients from many evolving perspectives on the brain *and* the mind.

The importance of keeping this open ear to the widest range of theories and treatment modalities is evident in thinking about Oliver, Maria and Samuel. To conceive of their suffering either as the direct result of renegade chemical messengers in the brain or simply as the unfortunate outcome of painful life stories, would be to miss the more likely possibility that their disorders were *multifactorial*—that an unhealthy alliance of biological, genetic, social and psychological influences had combined to precipitate illness.

If Oliver, for example, had had less of a genetic tendency toward overactive dopaminergic brain cells *or* better parenting *or* more supports in the community *or* a daughter who was never romanced by California, perhaps he would have escaped his dramatic symptoms.

Maria might have been better able to withstand the stress of her grandson's departure had she been less socially isolated, less vulnerable biologically or, perhaps, less sensitized to abandonment by early life experiences.

Although Samuel's age and physical infirmity clearly put him at risk for delirium, his symptoms might have been dramatically different had he not been traumatized by Ned's death. Evaluating the possible roles of infection, medication toxicity and alcohol withdrawal was essential in treating his condition, but so was thinking about his life.

It is in writing a patient's *psychiatric formulation* that a psychiatrist can weave threads from several perspectives together into a cohesive explanation of that person's symptomatology. Here the sometimes unwieldy pieces of medical, genetic, social and psychological data gathered from the patient are synthesized into a comprehensive clinical story that leads naturally to possible diagnoses and treatments.

Every story, of course, has an author. The formulation I write of a patient can be colored not only by which schools of thought within psychiatry I find most compelling, but by which particular issues in the patient's life capture my attention. This editing is partly conscious and partly unconscious. Based on my own life experiences, I may resonate strongly with one developmental challenge, or one emotional theme, and not another.

A complete formulation, therefore, attempts to draw on several wells of organization and perspective:

1. ***Diagnostic and Statistical Manual* criteria** (as discussed in Chapters 3 and 5): The psychiatric formulation includes a consideration of how the patient's signs and symptoms can logically be grouped into one or more known DSM syndromes.
2. **The influence of bodily abnormalities and genetic predispositions:** How might physical infirmity, medication side effects or alcohol and drug use be reflected in the psychiatric symptoms at hand? Might the patient be at risk for pathology based on his or her genetic heritage?
3. **Psychosocial factors:** How might the patient's social circumstances be involved in his or her suffering? Is the patient isolated? Has he or she lost a job? What stresses are operating in his or her relationships?
4. **Psychological factors:** What is the coloring of the psychological screen onto which these biological, genetic and psychosocial influences are projected? What developmental events in the patient's life are crucial to an understanding of how he or she will react to the stresses at hand? What does his or her earlier life history predict about the way he or she will respond to job loss, a physical handicap, the end of a romance or the death of a loved one?

For any given patient, one influence may seem to dramatically outweigh others. In a patient who is depressed and is found to have a cancer of the pancreas (the depression then being formally called an "organic mood syndrome"), the cancer is considered the likely etiology of the psychiatric symptoms. But, even then, social circumstances and psychological factors will be crucial in assessing how the individual will cope with his or her illness. Pancreatic cancer to one person may irrationally represent retribution for past sins, while to another it may mean being unfairly cut short of a particular cherished goal.

Thinking About the Brain

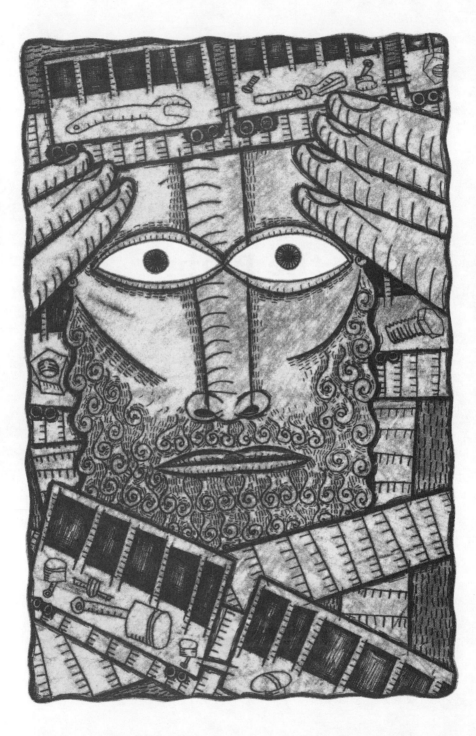

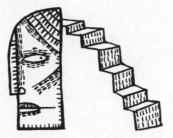

8

Broken

Nicholas seemed to fill the room where we met for the first time. A red flannel shirt strained to cover his shoulders. His huge hands, too big even for his bulky arms, testified that they had found a purpose in the world. There was grease in the crevices over his knuckles. Dried blood lined newer scratches, and numerous scars marked the old. His long, full beard was well trimmed and made him seem older than his thirty-two years.

His eyes made the walls seem close. They had been locked on mine almost constantly, hardly blinking, for the few minutes it took me to explain how his outpatient evaluation would proceed. The level of Nicholas's concentration made me overly conscious of what I was saying. After I had finished explaining how the clinic worked, I asked him to tell me what was troubling him. He stared at me several seconds, then nodded.

"I'm broken," he said, finally. His hands went up to his head, the thick fingers spread out on either side of his face. "Up here," he said. "Something's broken inside." He looked at me blankly.

"Broken?" I asked.

"Gear stuck, I figure." He pointed with one finger at the crown of his head, then let his hands relax on his thighs. "Gummed up. Has to be it,

Portions of this chapter were first published in *The Washington Post*.

seein' as I can't keep up at work anymore. The boss is about to fire me. And he's right to do it, too, because I'm broken down upstairs."

"What sort of work do you do?"

"I'm a mechanic," Nicholas said, smiling for the first time. "Not a *good* mechanic, either. I'm a *great* mechanic. I repair subway trains for the 'T.' You know, green line, red line, orange line . . ."

"Have you been at that job long?"

"Since, well . . . let's see . . . I don't want to be inaccurate here. You need the facts in order to fix me. I was three, maybe three-and-a-half months out from my nineteenth birthday. So, goin' on fourteen years. But it doesn't seem that long, except when I say it outright like that." Nicholas stared intently now and leaned forward. His voice choked with emotion. "I love those cars, the old ones especially. I can listen to one of those babies roll down Beacon Street and tell you which cylinder is bad. I can feel it. Eighty, ninety percent of the time I can tell you when a bearing's ready to go. Sometimes, it'll even wake me up in the middle of the night."

"You dream about your work . . . ?"

"No. Let's get this right, 'cause the way I figure I got no chance, otherwise. You're not gonna be able to get my gears in line if I don't give you the facts." He squinted. "See, I wake up 'cause I got a room directly where Route 9 turns into Huntington. Fifth floor, right over that sharp curve there. The cars slow down to make that curve, then speed up real quick. So I can hear the brakes, the wheels, the gearbox— the whole shebang—which is why I moved there in the first place. If somethin's way off, I wake up, look outside and grab the number off the train. I tell you, I'm on top of those cars even when I'm sleeping."

"What's the trouble at work?"

Nicholas shifted uncomfortably in his seat. "They say I'm slow."

"And what do you think?"

"I get stuck sometimes. I ain't slow. I just get so I can't move real quick. Sometimes I hear a train goin' down the track, and, if it's not just right, then, sure, I might spend some time—O.K., sometimes ten, maybe twelve hours—taking the engine apart, looking for what's causing a vibration or a ping. I might not go home that night. I might work through till the morning. Meanwhile, the other cars are piling up for repairs, and the boss is getting mad, which he should, saying it don't *matter* if there's a little vibration. Well, it might not matter to *him*, but it matters a whole hell of a lot to *me*. To him, maybe being a mechanic is just a job. To me, it's more than that. It's my life. It's like a religion." Nicholas slumped slightly in his seat. "But I can see his side of things, too. Which is why I'm here. I feel out of line. I want to keep my job. It's all I've got."

"You don't have other things in your life?"

"I don't want *other things*. Don't you *see*?" Nicholas strained to keep his frustration from turning to anger. He patted his thighs with those big hands and took a deep breath. "I don't *need* hobbies. I don't *need* a girl. I don't *need* a vacation. I have *engines*, and, if you *knew* engines, you'd know there's a whole world inside 'em. My God, a single piston can go wrong a dozen ways. Too much friction, too little friction, timing off, seal leak . . ."

I interrupted. "Nicholas, I understand what the engines mean to you." The intensity of his stare struck me, again. "I do understand," I said slowly. "Have you always been so involved with mechanics?"

"Don't get me wrong, I loved my work from day one. I don't want this misunderstood." His eyes misted over. "This year things finally snapped into place. Everything got clearer. I stopped wasting time. I worked twice as hard and twice as long. I moved to my room over the tracks. I think I learned as much about trains in the last ten months as I did the first twelve years on the job."

I was tempted to linger with the poetry in Nicholas's life—a man smitten with the engine, virtually *becoming* his craft. There was irrationality in his love, but there was also great commitment, a religious intensity and an undeniable beauty. Didn't I know, after all, what joy it was to have fallen in love with my own work?

Still, I had to agree with Nicholas, he seemed broken. His love had taken on pathologic proportions, isolating him and nearly costing him his job.

Much of what Nicholas was experiencing and exhibiting, in fact, can occur in patients suffering with epileptic seizures, particularly those affecting the brain's temporal lobes. Although the findings are controversial, researchers have noted that some of these patients share traits, including extreme emotional intensity, religiosity, changes in sexual appetite (usually reduced) and something called *viscosity*, or stickiness.

Epileptic seizures are caused by abnormal electrical discharges in the brain. Symptoms can be dramatic. Patients can lose consciousness completely while their limbs jerk wildly. Some simply become dazed, mute and immobile. In other cases, there are more subtle changes in behavior and emotion, without any alteration in the patient's level of consciousness. The changes can persist between seizures, as well.

The temporal lobes include what researchers consider the main emotional circuitry of the brain—the limbic system. One limbic structure, the amygdala, is thought to play a central role in directing emotions to appropriate targets. I wondered whether Nicholas's displacement of all his passion onto trains could really be the result of bad wiring in his amygdala.

The word "sticky" certainly fit. Nicholas hadn't, for a moment, allowed me to listen casually. His gaze was penetrating. His serious tone and unusual concern with detail demanded attention. He couldn't unglue himself from one engine in order to service others.

My suspicion doubled when Nicholas reported having been "knocked out" by a fall off a train platform about two years before. Head trauma, with resulting damage to the brain (such as scar tissue), can result in the runaway circuits of epilepsy.

The electroencephalogram (EEG) uses a series of sensitive paste-on electrodes, typically placed on the scalp or in nasal passages, to measure electrical activity in the brain. Nicholas's EEG showed abnormal discharges in his left temporal lobe.

I gave Nicholas the results of his EEG at our second meeting.

He was obviously relieved by the news. "So it ain't a bum gear. More like a cylinder misfirin'," he grinned. He looked up, as if trying to inspect his own brain. "How do we get at it?"

"I'd recommend you start taking a medicine called carbamazepine," I said. "It helps stop abnormal electrical activity in the brain."

"Well . . ." Nicholas pondered. He laced his fingers together and cracked his massive knuckles. "Let's get it tuned."

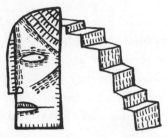

9

Alone With the Brain

Men ought to know that from nothing else but thence (from the brain) come joys, delights, laughter, and sports; and sorrows, griefs, despondency, and lamentations . . . by the same organ we become mad and delirious, and fears and terrors assail us, some by night and some by day. . . . All these things we endure from the brain when it is not healthy.

—Hippocrates

One of the reasons Nicholas's story remains vivid in my memory is that he sought me out with a complaint about his brain. No other patient had before, and none has since. This may seem trivial at first, but only because we expect psychiatric illness to weave itself nearly seamlessly into an individual's mental life. Whatever the role of disturbed brain chemistry or anatomy in producing an individual's symptoms, the usual onlooker's view of a sick body part—as in, "My leg hurts!"—is generally absent. The self may feel injured, the world may appear changed or bizarre or hostile, but the brain, under cover of its own pathology, somehow escapes anything more than vague suspicion.

From the outset, therefore, most patients interpret their psychiatric symptoms using life story reasoning. Themes prevail. Low mood at the leading edge of a depression doesn't prompt a person to question whether his or her neurotransmitters have run amuck; it moves that person to introspection or to a critical assessment of his or her environment. Patients come to psychiatrists already having constructed intuitive, but not always accurate or rational, story lines about why they feel the way they do.

The fact that most psychiatrists accept that electrical, chemical or structural brain abnormalities can be a crucial part of those stories initially puts us at a cognitive distance from our patients. We know, from the start, that treating the brain may turn out to be an important component of the therapy we offer.

Justifying our confidence can be difficult, because psychiatry still hasn't arrived at a point where we can definitively demonstrate the specific bodily abnormality responsible for a particular disorder or the exact mechanism by which our treatments correct it. Unlike doctors treating infectious disease, we can't isolate an offending bacterium and then watch it be destroyed by an antibiotic. Our evidence that medications and electroconvulsive therapy (ECT) are useful is largely *empirical*—based on clinical trials in which patients with a given diagnosis suffer less after receiving the treatment under study.

Faced with unwieldy gaps in our knowledge about the brain, yet educated to link symptoms to bodily abnormalities, we have been understandably romanced by the facts at hand. We have allowed the comforting public perceptions that a "chemical imbalance" *causes* schizophrenia and that depression is "inherited," when the discoveries underlying such catchphrases are, in fact, fascinating and useful pieces of a very unfinished puzzle.

The following pages outline the basic anatomy and physiology necessary to appreciate the real power and promise of psychiatry's new treatments. It is not my hope that reading them will allow you to package psychiatric illness into neat biochemical bundles. To the contrary, I would have you struggle, as I have struggled, to understand and accept the ambiguities and mysteries inherent in a field on the frontier of the body's most complex organ.

Wet Circuits

The communication system of the brain is made up of over 100 billion electrochemical cells called *neurons*. Like wires in a staggering telephone network, each cell is able to receive chemical messages from up to 200,000 other neurons and to distribute its own signal to hundreds more.

After receiving so many messages, a neuron has only one decision to make—whether or not to *fire* an electrical charge down its long *axon*. When the charge is fired, the effect is to release the cell's own chemical messengers from a collection of tiny sacs, called *vesicles*, in its terminal end (Figure 1).

There are many known chemical messengers, called *neurotransmitters*, which are essentially the languages spoken between one neuron and another (Figure 2). Some exhort their target cells to fire, whereas others urge them to remain quiet. The method by which a nerve cell integrates so many disparate communications is one of the great unknowns of the nervous system.

Neurotransmitters are synthesized from amino-acid building blocks within neurons. The reactions that produce them would proceed at a snail's pace were it not for enzyme catalysts that greatly speed up each biochemical step. In an elegant display of biological economy, one neurotransmitter is often the raw material for another.

In order to exert its effect, a neurotransmitter must flow across a fluid-filled space between the "speaking" neuron and the "listening" neuron (Figure 3). This is a journey across vigorous tides. The gap to be traversed (the *synaptic cleft*) contains enzymes responsible for breaking down the neurotransmitters when they are done delivering their mes-

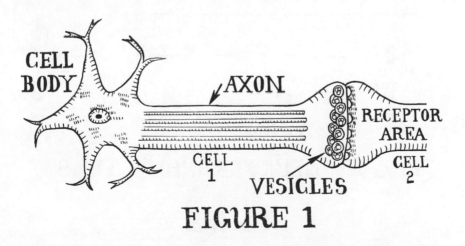

FIGURE 1

sages. What's more, in what amounts to a cellular undertow (called *reuptake*), the speaking neuron can reabsorb and inactivate the neurotransmitters it has just released. Both processes are essential to control the final volume of the chemical information transferred.

Even once the synaptic cleft has been crossed, neurotransmitters cannot be "heard" until they attach to specialized ears, called *receptors*, on the listening neuron. There are different kinds of receptors, and each will accommodate only one kind of neurotransmitter. The neurotransmitter dopamine, for example, is effectively mute until it finds and attaches to specialized dopamine receptors.

The *synapse* is the principal military theater for psychiatry's pharmacologic war on illness. Extremely effective medications have been developed which can selectively enhance or diminish the activity of a given neurotransmitter. This can be achieved in any one of several ways—by increasing its production, promoting or interfering with its release, preventing its inactivation (by hindering the reuptake system or the synaptic cleft enzymes), or blocking access to its target receptors (Figure 4).

The rationale for sculpting the wet circuits of the brain in these ways comes from theories that mental illnesses such as schizophrenia, depres-

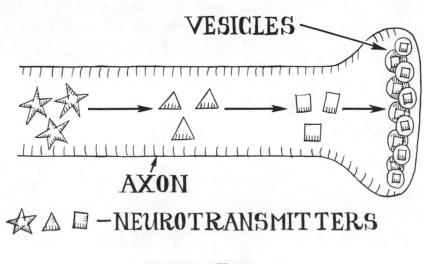

FIGURE 2

sion, and panic disorder are due, wholly or in part, to the relative over-abundance or deficiency of one or more neurotransmitters.

Extrapolating from synapses and neurotransmitters to thought and perception would be a momentous intellectual leap. Psychiatry is not on the brink of making it. Using television as an analogy for the brain, we have learned that manipulating the antenna in particular ways improves reception, but we don't know precisely why. We have even less insight into how the antenna could be linked to the *content* of the dramas unfolding on screen.

The Vulnerable Brain

With over 100 billion electrically and chemically connected cells, the brain is primed for chaos. The blood vessels carrying its oxygen and other nutrients can burst, leak or become blocked. Toxins can reach and accumulate in its tissues, causing immediate or delayed injury. Electrical circuits can discharge haphazardly (as in Nicholas's case), spilling neurotransmitters.

The brain also sits in precarious surroundings. Although the skull offers some protection from trauma, it does so at the price of confining the brain

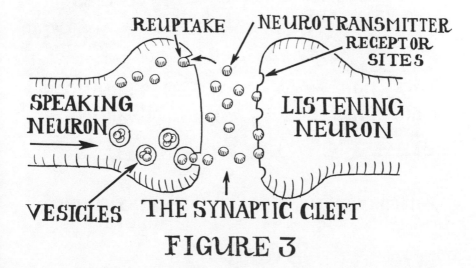

FIGURE 3

within its rigid walls. This makes the brain particularly sensitive to pathologic processes—whether a bleed, infection or tumor—that compete for space. It also makes it hostage to choking pressure should the normal flow of cerebrospinal fluid between its tissues and the spinal cord be blocked.

The brain is not a homogeneous network of neurons. The neurons are organized into discrete, interconnected structures with specific functions. The occipital lobes, for instance, process visual information. The thalamus is intimately involved in the perception of pain. The hippocampus plays an essential role in memory.

Organic mental disorders—those disorders with readily identifiable bodily causes—tell us a great deal about the changes in thought, perception and behavior that can result from particular disruptions in and around brain tissue. Some of these bodily causes, by interfering with metabolism (e.g., thyroid disease) or blood flow (e.g., massive heart attack), seem to affect the brain as a whole, whereas others (e.g., temporal lobe seizures) cause more localized disturbance.

Psychiatrists want to make certain that no reversible bodily cause of a patient's suffering goes undetected. We keep careful watch, therefore,

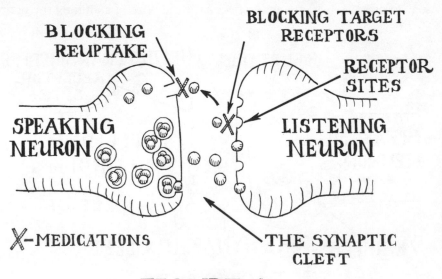

FIGURE 4

for the signs and symptoms of neurological impairment. Although an exhaustive list of organic mental disorders would be unwieldy, sampling the brain's connections with behavior and emotion should convince us of the mysteries and potentials within psychiatry's domain.

The Frontal Lobes

The two frontal lobes of the brain (left and right), which play major roles in both emotion and body movement, sit highest in the skull, just behind the brow (Figure 5).

A lesion, such as a bleed or tumor, in this area can lead to dramatic changes in personality and behavior. Often the personality is unleashed, *disinhibited* in psychiatric parlance, and the individual becomes over-familiar and tactless and talks too much.

Damage to the frontal lobes even puts one's moral fiber in jeopardy. Victims can become euphoric, impulsive, profane and demanding. They can lose the ability to empathize with the suffering of others and to feel remorse. Gross errors in judgment, sometimes leading to sexual indiscretions or financial risk taking, are not unusual.

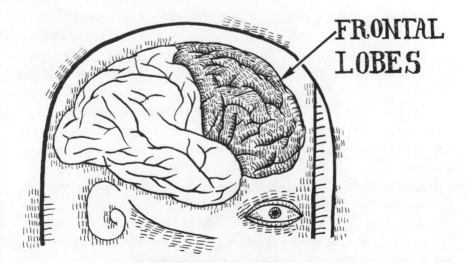

FRONTAL LOBES

FIGURE 5

In 1848, the physician J. M. Harlow wrote of his patient Phineas Gage, a foreman injured when a crowbar penetrated his frontal lobes:

> He is fitful, irreverent, indulging at times in the grossest profanity (which was not previously his custom), manifesting but little deference to his fellows, impatient of restraint or advice when it conflicts with his desires, at times pertinaciously obstinate yet capricious and vascillating [sic], devising many plans for future operation which are no sooner arranged than they are abandoned in turn for others appearing more feasible. . . . His mind was radically changed, so that his friends and acquaintances said he was no longer Gage.

Oliver Sacks, in his book *The Man Who Mistook His Wife for a Hat*, described a patient of his own who suffered with multiple sclerosis affecting her frontal lobes:

> She speaks very quickly, impulsively, and (it seems) indifferently . . . so that the important and the trivial, the true and the false, the serious and the joking, are poured out in rapid, unselective, half-confabulatory stream. . . . She may contradict herself within a few seconds . . . will say she loves music, she doesn't, she has a broken hip, she hasn't . . .

Many frontal lobe symptoms, it should not be missed, mimic those of mania. Here, then, is a call to the physicianly art of differential diagnosis. The biological cynicism cultivated in medical school, the tendency to second-guess oneself and one's colleagues, the contempt for simple answers must all be brought to bear. Rushing to a diagnosis of mania, invoking a compelling life story to turn such suffering to poetry, even being satisfied prescribing a drug like lithium, might doom a patient who could otherwise have had a growing and benign tumor successfully removed.

There is much room for wonder here, too, because some frontal lobe patients, far from falling victim to disinhibition, become apathetic, withdrawn and slow to move (a syndrome which can be mistaken for depression). Some patients become demented, others lose the capacity for abstract reasoning and problem solving, and still others retain their intellect.

Even massive lesions in the frontal lobes can go undetected for years, causing only subtle personality changes. No one understands precisely why. And no one can explain exactly why it is that intrusive, insensitive, seemingly amoral individuals often would turn out to have, in the eyes of our current testing methods, perfectly normal-looking frontal lobes.

The Parietal Lobes

The two parietal lobes are located just behind the frontal lobes, under the crown of the skull (Figure 6). Damage here, whether by injury or illness, can cause a bewildering array of disabilities.

Vision can become useless in judging distances and dimensions. Spatial orientation and memory can be impaired to such an extent that a patient may be unable to locate a well-known room on the ward, or even become lost in the familiar surroundings of home.

The ability to recognize objects by touch, something we do automatically each time we reach into pockets for keys or change, can be so

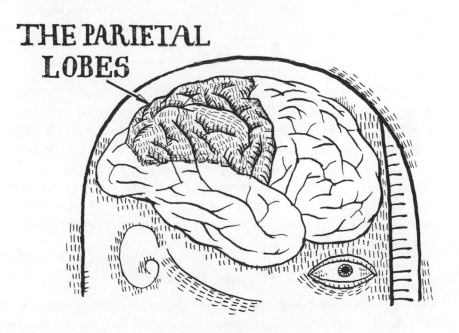

THE PARIETAL LOBES

FIGURE 6

impaired that a patient, while blindfolded, will be baffled as to whether a quarter or a penny has just been placed in his or her hand.

Particularly important for psychiatry is that profoundly depressed mood, accompanied by psychosis, has been known to occur in patients with parietal lobe injuries, especially if a stroke has damaged the right lobe.

Occasionally, body image becomes grossly distorted. Patients disown arms or legs, insisting that their own extremities do not exist or that they belong to someone else. Even more rarely, an individual with a parietal lobe lesion may believe he or she has extra body parts, such as two left arms.

The researcher N. Lukianowicz recollected one patient's description of the following symptoms consistent with parietal lobe epilepsy:

> I get the feeling in my eyes that they tear out of their sockets, and rush out from the cabin, till they touch the people and the houses and the lamp-posts along the road. . . . Then everything rushes towards me again and my eyeballs hurry back into their sockets. At other times I might feel my hands and arms grow long very rapidly, till they seem to reach miles ahead. A moment later they begin to shrink until they come back to their normal size. I may have such a feeling several times in a minute or two.

Again, the medical training of psychiatrists looms large. The signs and symptoms of parietal lobe stroke, for example, can look like those of Alzheimer's disease, major depression or a delusional disorder. A naive clinician, jumping prematurely to one of these diagnoses, might be satisfied when antidepressant and antipsychotic medications improve the patient's mental status. But this apparent therapeutic success would be a tragic diversion if it obscured the real culprit, such as untreated hypertension or an infected heart valve, either of which could go on to cause a second stroke.

The Corpus Callosum

The two hemispheres of the brain communicate with one another via a thick band of neurons running side to side, called the corpus callosum (Figure 7). If this connection is disrupted (by a tumor, for instance), the brain is essentially split down the middle.

A number of *disconnection* syndromes have been described in the scientific literature. Some include personality changes or psychotic symptoms. One of the most dramatic is called *alien hand*. In this syndrome, the patient is unshakably convinced that one hand, usually the left, has a will of its own. It is capable of gentleness or violence, creativity or destruction. It can even attack the rest of the body.

When a patient reports a symptom like alien hand, his or her therapist might be moved to interpret it entirely symbolically, rather than neurologically. If the patient speaks, for example, of having been abused *at the hand* of his father, it would be tempting to interpret alien hand as the embodiment of that abuse. While appealing thematically, however, this life story reasoning should never preclude a thorough search for underlying organic pathology. As did Nicholas's epilepsy, the alien hand reminds us of the imperative of thinking about the brain, even as we keep an ear open to the poetry of the mind.

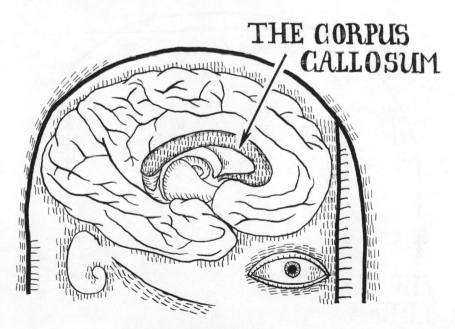

THE CORPUS CALLOSUM

FIGURE 7

The Temporal Lobes

As mentioned before, the temporal lobes (Figure 8), located at the base of the brain, contain several components of what is known as the *limbic system*. The limbic system is a far-reaching network of connected brain structures that share common neurotransmitters and seem to play a powerful role in memory, emotion and motivated behaviors such as eating and mating. The structures have names like the amygdala, hippocampus, cingulate gyrus, thalamus and hypothalamus.

Injury to some limbic structures seems to result in increased aggression, whereas injury elsewhere brings passivity. In experiments conducted with monkeys, damage to the amygdala and area immediately surrounding it resulted in vastly increased sexual activity and unusual friendliness toward human beings.

Nicholas's case dramatizes the personality changes, including obsessiveness, that can result from a seizure disorder involving the temporal

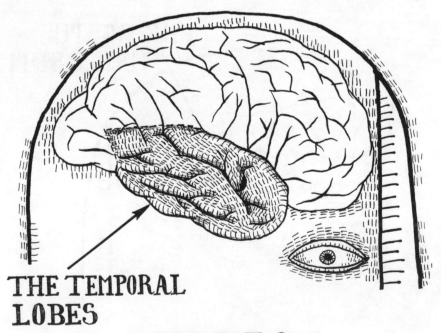

THE TEMPORAL
LOBES

FIGURE 8

lobes. Disease here (whether epilepsy, infection, tumor or stroke) can also cause impaired speech, increased or decreased mood, altered sex drive, paranoia or hallucinations.

The neurologist Marsel Mesulam described another patient with temporal lobe epilepsy who complained of sudden mood swings:

> She reported feeling intensely depressed and tearful when listening to a certain piece of dance music. Since the music did not sound particularly moody to other observers, and since it was not associated with any particularly sad event in her life, an electroencephalogram (EEG) was obtained while she was listening to it. The onset of music was associated with intense EEG spike discharges [i.e., seizure activity], depression, and crying. There were no other sensory, motor, or autonomic manifestations of epilepsy. At least some of the mood swings in this patient could therefore be explained on the basis of complex reflex epilepsy.

Occipital Lobes

The occipital lobes, which process the visual information received by the eyes, are located at the back of the brain (Figure 9). As might be expected, damage to this area can result in visual distortions, hallucinations and blindness.

The content of the distortions and hallucinations can be influenced by an individual's emotional and intellectual history. A person who was assaulted as a child, for example, might "see" acts of violence being committed, rather than seeing strange animals.

This speaks directly to psychiatry's proper role at the interface of the brain and the mind. When an otherwise healthy patient reports the onset of visual hallucinations, the necessity for a neurological workup is clear. To do less would be to ignore the fact that bodily abnormalities often cause psychiatric symptoms. But even the discovery of an occipital lobe tumor does not relieve us from attempting to understand the *meaning* of the hallucinations to the individual. To do less would be to ignore the fact that patients become ill *in their own ways*. Lessening their pain demands that we hear their symptoms in the context of their life stories.

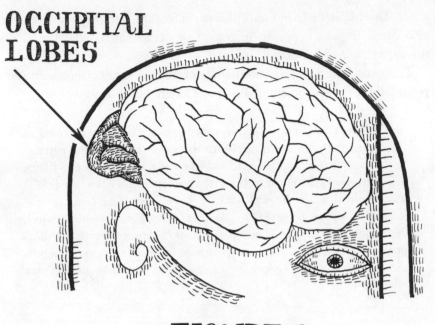

OCCIPITAL
LOBES

FIGURE 9

Windows on the Brain

For hundreds of years, physicians have attempted to visualize and document the workings of the brain. Among the first was Franz Joseph Gall, a Viennese physiologist who lived from 1758 to 1828. Gall postulated that the brain was divided into 27 different organs, each with a different function (Figure 10). These organs corresponded to bumps in various locations on the surface of the head. Mental disorders, therefore, could be identified by irregularities in the terrain of the skull, the mapping and study of which was called *phrenology*.

Phrenology did not survive scientific scrutiny, but Gall's idea that parts of the brain had specific functions was borne out. Our technologies for imaging the brain's various structures, measuring their metabolism and recording their electrical activities are direct descendants of Gall's intuitions.

Today, we have several windows on the brain. One of the most commonly used is the CAT scan. CAT stands for *computerized axial tomogra-*

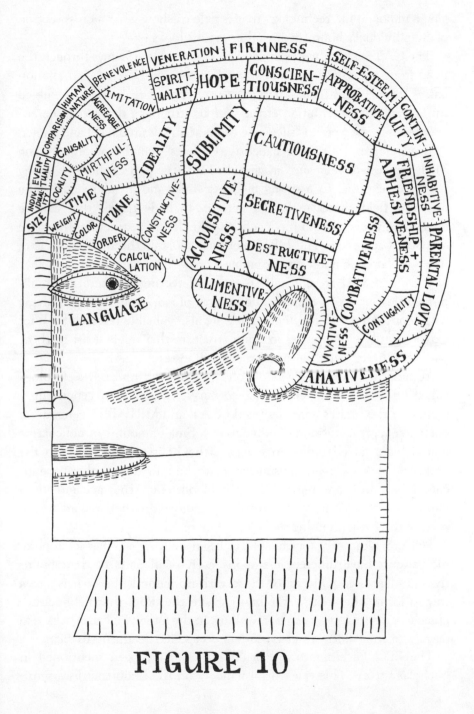

FIGURE 10

phy, a radiographic technology that is able to show what a cross section of an individual's brain (or any other organ) looks like.

The CAT scanner works by sending conventional X-rays through the head from many different angles and measuring how much radiation passes through the tissues along the way. The data is then assembled into a visual representation of the various structures that would be encountered if one were to "slice" the brain at any desired level and angle.

Even clearer (but more expensive) "slices" can be obtained using MRI, or *magnetic resonance imaging*. In MRI, the part of the body being studied is exposed to a strong magnetic field and a radio signal. The magnetic field causes molecular activity in body tissues that can be measured by receptors in the machine. The denser a structure, the more activity is recorded. The MRI machine tabulates the differences and, like CAT, uses computers to assemble a cross-sectional picture.

CAT and MRI are clinically useful in detecting structural brain abnormalities such as a tumor, collection of blood, or an area of scarring within or adjacent to the brain. They are also valuable research tools for exploring subtle differences in brain structure that might exist in those patients suffering with particular mental illnesses.

Yet another promising window on the brain is a research technology called PET, or *positron-emission tomography*. Rather than generating a picture of the brain's anatomy (as do CAT and MRI), PET generates a computer representation of brain activity. Small amounts of radioactive material are added either to glucose (the brain's main fuel), to the building blocks of neurotransmitters or to investigational pharmaceuticals. When these are injected into the bloodstream, they accumulate in various brain structures. A sensitive detector can then record which parts of the brain are using the injected materials.

PET provides a way, for example, to begin studying whether schizophrenic patients have different metabolic activity in parts of their brains than do depressed patients, or those with no mental illness. It is also a way to locate the areas of the brain where the drugs that fight schizophrenia or depression are actually working. In the future, PET may help us to diagnose mental illnesses and to better target specific treatments to them.

The EEG, or *electroencephalogram*, has already been mentioned in Nicholas's story. This is a crucial window on the brain that uses sensitive paste-on detectors to record the brain's electrical activity. Because very subtle seizures can cause a wide range of psychiatric symptoms, the EEG is a common component of a complete psychiatric assessment.

Finally, psychiatrists can gather information by studying the chemistry of several bodily fluids. One of the most important is *cerebrospinal fluid,* the substance that bathes the spinal cord and fills the hollow ventricles of the brain. Cerebrospinal fluid can be sampled (by performing a relatively simple procedure called a *lumbar puncture*) and tested for evidence of infection or other chemical abnormalities. Because the brain and spinal cord are metabolically linked with other organ systems, we can also collect essential data by studying a patient's blood or urine.

The Brain/Mind Problem

This book contains separate sections on the brain and the mind because explanations of psychological suffering and mental illness have tended to focus either on one or the other. Some psychiatrists, in fact, have chosen sides, maintaining either that all human interactions will eventually be understood in terms of brain chemistry and anatomy, or that such neurological reasoning is merely a distraction from the real challenge of understanding emotional dynamics.

In truth, neither perspective is about to replace the other. The power in psychiatry lies in allowing our understandings of the brain and the mind to coexist, to be used together in service to patients.

In reading the chapters that follow, I hope you will think frequently about Oliver, Maria, Samuel and Nicholas. You will find that their experiences with mental illness are not completely captured by any symptom list or scientific theory. This is because each person was truly ill in his or her own way. Each needed a psychiatry courageous enough not to choose sides, one that was willing to embrace the best of both medical model and life story reasoning.

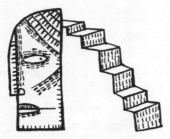

10

Schizophrenia

The Widow

Emil Kraepelin, who lived from 1856 to 1926, is considered the father of modern psychiatric diagnosis and classification. A German psychiatrist, he was the first to differentiate manic and depressive disorders from schizophrenia, which he called dementia praecox. *"The Widow" is one of his classic case histories of schizophrenia:*

The widow, aged thirty-five, whom I will now bring before you . . . gives full information about her life in answer to our questions, knows where she is, can tell the date and the year, and gives proof of satisfactory school knowledge. It is noteworthy that she does not look at her questioner, and speaks in a low and peculiar, sugary, affected tone. When you touch on her illness, she is reserved at first, and says that she is quite well, but she soon begins to express a number of remarkable *ideas of persecution.* For many years she has heard voices, which insult her and cast suspicion on her chastity. They mention a number of names she knows, and tell her she will be stripped and abused. The voices are very distinct, and, in her opinion, they must be carried by a telescope or a machine from her home. Her thoughts are dictated to her; she is obliged to think them, and hears them repeated after her. She is interrupted in her work, and has all kinds of uncomfortable sensations in her body, to which something is "done." In particular, her "mother parts" are turned inside out, and people send a pain through her back, lay ice-water on her heart, squeeze her neck, injure her spine, and violate her. There are also hallucinations of sight—black figures and the altered appearance of people—but these are far less frequent. She cannot exactly say who carries on all the influencing, or for what object it is done. Sometimes it is the people from her home, and sometimes the doctors of an asylum where she was before who have taken something out of her body.

The patient makes these extraordinary complaints without showing much emotion. She cries a little, but then describes her morbid experiences again with secret satisfaction and even with an erotic bias. She demands her discharge, but is easily consoled, and does not trouble at all about her position and her future. Her use of numerous strained and hardly intelligible phrases is very striking. She is ill-treated "flail-wise," "utterance-wise," "terror-wise"; she is "a picture of misery in angel's form," and "a defrauded mamma and housewife of sense of order." They have "altered her form of emotion." She is "persecuted by a secret insect from the District Office." . . .

. . . Her former history shows that she has been ill for nearly ten years. The disease developed gradually. About a year after the death of her husband, by whom she has two children, she became apprehensive, slept badly, heard loud talking in her room at night, and thought that she was being robbed of her means and persecuted by people from Frankfort, where she had formerly lived. Four years ago she spent a year in an asylum. She thought she found the "Frankforters" there, noticed poison in the food, heard voices, and felt influences. After her discharge she brought accusations against the doctors of having mutilated her while she was there. She now thought them to be her persecutors, and openly abused the public authorities for failing to protect her, so she had to be admitted to this hospital two months ago. Here she made the same complaints day after day, without showing much excitement, and wrote long-winded letters full of senseless and unvarying abuse about the persecution from which she suffered, to her relations, the asylum doctors, and the authorities. She did not occupy herself in any way, held no intercourse with her fellow-patients, and avoided every attempt to influence her.

Signs and Symptoms

In 1911, the Swiss psychiatrist Eugen Bleuler coined the term *schizophrenia* from the Greek words for split and mind. Like Kraepelin's widow, patients with this disorder seem to be split between reality and fantasy.

Plagued by hallucinations and delusions, they find it difficult to determine whether what they think, see and hear is real or "in their heads."

Over four million Americans are thought to be at risk for schizophrenia. Approximately 1 percent of the population will develop it at some point during their lives. The illness usually strikes between the ages of fifteen and thirty-five. Overall, it affects men as often as it does women, but men seem to fall victim at a younger age.

Schizophrenia tends to begin gradually with a prodromal phase of the illness that can linger for months.[†] The earliest signs and symptoms include social isolation, feelings of anxiety, lack of energy and loss of concentration.

Invariably, the patient's level of functioning deteriorates. This may be evident in decreased performance at work, less interest in personal hygiene or trouble maintaining relationships.

An active phase of the illness, marked by psychotic symptoms, follows the prodromal, or precursory, phase. The most common psychotic symptom is auditory hallucinations (hearing voices). Frequently, the patient hears a voice commenting on his or her behavior or thoughts. In other cases, the patient overhears two or more voices talking with each other.

Visual hallucinations (seeing things), olfactory hallucinations (smelling things) and tactile hallucinations (feeling things on one's body) also occur in the active phase of schizophrenia, but less often.

Patients commonly suffer with delusions (fixed false beliefs). Some believe that they are being stalked, or that people close to them have been unfaithful and are untrustworthy. They may insist that their thoughts are being stolen, broadcast to others or inserted in their minds by unfriendly forces.

Alternatively, the psychosis can center on a part of the patient's body. He or she may actually *feel* a bodily organ rotting away (a *somatic hallucination*) or believe that a snake lives in his or her bloodstream (a *somatic delusion*).

[†]The complete DSM-III-R diagnostic criteria for schizophrenia can be found in Appendix E.

Thought processes can become markedly disordered, so that the patient stops making any sense at all, rattling off ideas that have no obvious relationship to one another (*loosening of associations*).

Emotions may seem to wither. The patient's face may become nearly expressionless (*blunted* or *flat affect*). Alternatively, his or her emotional reactions may become grossly exaggerated and inappropriate.

A diagnosis of schizophrenia is only made once the condition has lasted six months and included the active, psychotic phase. When symptoms disappear sooner, a diagnosis of *schizophreniform disorder* is made.

Different types of schizophrenia have been identified. In the *catatonic* type, the primary feature of the illness is that the patient's movements and level of activity have changed dramatically. He or she may become rigid, may maintain strange postures or may constantly move about without any clear purpose.

Paranoid schizophrenia is marked by the patient's mistaken belief (sometimes reinforced by the content of auditory hallucinations) that he or she is being persecuted.

Disorganized schizophrenia is diagnosed when the dominant signs of the illness are incoherence, purposeless behavior or blunted affect. Some patients seem childish or silly.

The symptoms of schizophrenia tend to fluctuate as the illness shifts from its active phase to a simmering residual phase, then back again. Residual symptoms can last years, and include poor hygiene, lack of energy, depressed mood, odd beliefs (e.g., in black magic or clairvoyance) and peculiar behavior (e.g., talking to oneself in public or hoarding food).

Over the course of the illness, the active symptoms, such as hallucinations, usually become less intense. The residual symptoms, however, may worsen.

The prognosis for recovery from schizophrenia is best when the illness begins abruptly following a known emotional stressor, such as the loss of a loved one. As troubling as they can be at the time, overt ("positive") signs and symptoms—including changes in mood and the presence of anxiety, hostility, confusion and psychosis—actually predict a less severe long-term course of the illness. Poorer prognosis is associated with a gradual onset of illness that occurs without a known stressor.

It is also foreshadowed by the persistence of the less overt, more muted ("negative") symptoms of schizophrenia, such as social withdrawal and blunted affect.

In addition, patients with the paranoid and catatonic types of schizophrenia are thought to fare better than those with the disorganized type.

Although schizophrenia was once considered a uniformly chronic illness that worsened inexorably over time, it is now believed that, with treatment, as many as a third of patients go on to lead fairly normal lives. Another third continue to struggle with significant symptoms but function reasonably well in the community. The last third, unfortunately, remain seriously impaired and require frequent (or chronic) hospitalizations.

Is Schizophrenia Inherited?

There is now a good deal of scientific data to back up Emil Kraepelin's clinical impression that a vulnerability to schizophrenia is inherited. In 1907, he wrote that "defective heredity is a very prominent factor . . . in the illness."

Recent research has shown that children with one schizophrenic parent have more than ten times the risk of developing the illness than do children in the general population. If both parents are schizophrenic, the risk may be as high as fifty times the normal risk. Even if these children are adopted and raised by parents without the illness, the increased risk persists.

Brothers and sisters of someone with schizophrenia also have a much greater likelihood of developing it. What's more, when schizophrenia strikes siblings, it often begins at approximately the same age in each.

Studies of identical twins add more evidence. If one identical twin suffers from schizophrenia, there is a 50 to 60 percent chance that the other twin will also be affected. This is true even if the twins are raised in separate households.

If schizophrenia were a purely genetic illness, we might expect that identical twins, whose genes are exactly the same, would always share the illness. The fact that they don't indicates that other variables, perhaps environmental ones, must be involved in determining whether symptoms develop.

Schizophrenia and the Brain

The specific neurological causes of schizophrenia remain unknown. Researchers do, however, have several hypotheses. One revolves around the idea that schizophrenic symptoms might be the result of overactivity of a neurotransmitter called *dopamine*, which is particularly abundant in the limbic system. This theory is supported by the fact that drugs which increase dopamine activity—including cocaine, amphetamine and a medication called L-dopa (used to treat Parkinson's disease)—can bring about or worsen psychosis. It is also consistent with the finding that the antipsychotic medications that are used to control schizophrenia block receptors for dopamine in the brain. In fact, the more powerful a medicine is as a dopamine blocker, the more effective it is at relieving psychosis.

Imbalances of other neurotransmitters, including norepinephrine, gamma-aminobutyric acid (GABA) and serotonin, have also been implicated in schizophrenia.

Brain imaging techniques such as CAT, MRI and PET (see Chapter 9) have been used to determine whether there are structural or metabolic differences between the brains of schizophrenic patients and those of people who do not suffer from the illness. Such techniques have revealed that, in a percentage of schizophrenic patients, parts of the brain involved in complex thought processes (including an area called the *prefrontal cortex*) have atrophied or developed abnormally. In contrast, the brain's hollow, fluid-filled ventricles are often enlarged. Blood flow and metabolism, particularly in the frontal and parietal lobes, are often abnormal, as well.

Because many schizophrenic patients were born in late winter or early spring, some scientists have theorized that the illness may be seeded when mothers are infected with a virus during the winter months of their pregnancies.

Others have noted that schizophrenia has features in common with autoimmune disorders, in which infection-fighting cells attack the body itself. Like lupus, for example, schizophrenia develops most commonly during adolescence or young adulthood, worsens and improves in cycles, and runs in families. These similarities raise the question of whether schizophrenia might result when the immune system attacks certain parts of the brain.

Most researchers agree, however, that schizophrenia is probably not caused by any one factor. More likely is that certain individuals are biologically predisposed to the illness, symptoms of which are then triggered by a wide variety of possible emotional or physical stressors. This is another way of saying that psychiatry continues to embrace a vision of this major mental illness as some unhealthy alliance between the brain and the mind.

Medicines for Schizophrenia

Antipsychotic (or *neuroleptic*) medications, first introduced in the 1950s, significantly reduce psychotic symptoms in as many as 75 percent of the schizophrenic patients who receive them. These agents are also very effective in preventing relapse from the residual phase of the illness to the active phase.

The antipsychotics vary in structure, potency and side effects (see Table 10–1), but each of them seems to work by blocking dopamine

Table 10–1. Antipsychotic medications

| | | Side effects | | |
Trade name	Generic name	Sedation	Movement/ muscular	Low blood pressure
Thorazine	Chlorpromazine	More	Medium	Medium
Vesprin	Triflupromazine	Medium	More	Medium
Mellaril	Thioridazine	More	Less	Medium
Trilafon	Perphenazine	Medium	Medium	Less
Stelazine	Trifluoperazine	Less	More	Less
Prolixin	Fluphenazine	Less	More	Less
Tindal	Acetophenazine	Medium	Medium	Less
Navane	Thiothixene	Less	More	Less
Taractan	Chlorprothixene	More	Medium	Medium
Haldol	Haloperidol	Less	More	Less
Moban	Molindone	Medium	Less	Much less
Loxitane	Loxapine	Medium	Medium	Less
Orap	Pimozide	Less	More	Less

receptors in the brain. Unfortunately, this dopamine blockade can also cause disturbances of movement, including muscle spasms, muscular rigidity, tremor, facial tics and intense restlessness.

Sometimes these side effects can be avoided or limited by finding an antipsychotic that seems to "agree" with the patient, and then using the lowest effective dosage. A number of supplementary medications are also available which, used in conjunction with antipsychotics, help to maintain more normal muscle tone and function.

One particularly troubling movement disorder linked to the use of antipsychotics is called *tardive dyskinesia*. This condition, particularly common in the elderly, begins with uncontrollable movements of the mouth and tongue that are irreversible in the majority of cases. It can progress to involve the extremities, neck and shoulders. Between 20 and 30 percent of schizophrenic patients treated for years with antipsychotics eventually develop the condition.

Unfortunately, antipsychotics block other neurotransmitters, including *acetylcholine* and *norepinephrine*. This can result in dry mouth, constipation, blurred vision, abnormal urination, glaucoma and problems with blood pressure. Supplementary medicines are often used to control these side effects, as well.

The newest antipsychotic is clozapine (trade name, Clozaril). Clozapine is remarkably effective in treating some patients with severe schizophrenia resistant to other antipsychotic medications. Its drawbacks include the fact that it can cause a potentially fatal shortage of white blood cells, called *agranulocytosis*. For this reason, its use is carefully monitored with frequent blood tests.

Despite the potential complications of treatment with antipsychotic medications, countless patients have been helped by them.

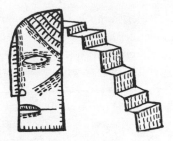

11

Mood Disorders

The Farmer

In another of Emil Kraepelin's classic clinical histories, "The Farmer," he describes a dramatic case of major depression:

I will place before you a farmer, aged fifty-nine, who was admitted to the hospital a year ago. The patient looks much older than he really is, principally owing to the loss of teeth from his upper jaw. He not only understands our questions without any difficulty, but answers them relevantly and correctly; can tell where he is, and how long he has been here; knows the doctors, and can give the date and the day of the week. His expression is dejected. The corners of his mouth are rather drawn down, and his eyebrows drawn together. . . . On being questioned about his illness, he breaks into lamentations, saying that he did not tell the whole truth on his admission, but concealed the fact that he had fallen into sin in his youth and practiced uncleanness with himself; everything he did was wrong. "I am so apprehensive, so wretched; I cannot lie still for anxiety. O God, if I had only not transgressed so grievously!" He has been ill for over a year, has had giddiness and headaches. It began with stomach-aches and head troubles, and he could not work any longer. "There was no impulse left." He can get no rest now, and fancies silly things, as if someone were in the room. Once it seemed to him that he had seen the Evil One: perhaps he would be carried off. So things seemed to him. As a boy, he had taken apples and nuts. "Conscience has said that that is not right; conscience has only awakened just now in my illness." He had also played with a cow, and by himself. "I reproach myself for that now." It seemed to him that he had fallen away from God. . . . His appetite is bad, and he has no stools. He cannot sleep. "If the mind does not sleep, all sorts of thoughts come." . . . He fastened his neckerchief to strangle himself, but he was not really in earnest. Three sisters and a brother were ill too. The sisters were not so bad; they soon recovered. . . .

The patient tells us this in broken sentences, interrupted by wailing and groaning. In all other respects, he behaves naturally, does whatever he is told, and only begs us not to let him be dragged away—"There is terrible apprehension in my heart." Except for a little trembling of the outspread fingers and slightly arhythmic [sic] action of the heart, we find no striking disturbances at the physical examination. As for the patient's former history, he is married, and has four healthy children, while three are dead. The illness began gradually seven or eight months before his admission, without any assignable cause. Loss of appetite and dyspepsia [upset stomach] appeared first, and then ideas of sin. . . .

The Spectrum of Mood Disorders

The farmer's illness, major depression, is one of several related *mood* (i.e., *affective*) *disorders*. Each of these conditions is marked by a prominent disturbance of mood—whether sadness, elation or alternating periods of each.

The suffering Kraepelin wrote of has also been described eloquently by a number of the artists who have fallen victim to affective disorders.[†] Gustav Mahler, the great composer, wrote to a childhood friend of his struggle with mood swings:

> Much has happened within me since my last letter; I cannot describe it. Only this: I have become a different person. I don't know whether this new person is better, he certainly is not happier. The fires of a supreme zest for living and the most gnawing desire for death alternate in my heart, sometimes in the course of a single hour. I know only one thing: I cannot go on like this!

[†]Passages by Gustav Mahler and Virginia Woolf quoted in J. R. DePaulo, K. R. Ablow: *How to Cope With Depression: A Complete Guide for You and Your Family*. New York, Ballantine Fawcett-Crest, 1991

The novelist Virginia Woolf shared her experience with the depression that ultimately led to her suicide:

> It strikes me—what are these sudden fits of complete exhaustion? I come in here to write; can't even finish a sentence; and am pulled under; now is this some odd effort; the subconscious pulling me down into her? I've been reading Faber on Newman; compared his account of a nervous breakdown; the refusal of some part of the mechanism; is that what happens to me? Not quite. Because I'm not evading anything. I long to write *The Pargiters*. No. I think the effort to live in two spheres: the novel and life; is a strain. . . . To have to behave with circumspection and decision to strangers wrenches me into another region; hence the collapse.

Such passages make clear that the pervasive mood disturbances outlined in the pages that follow are no close cousins of typical sadness and happiness. Unlike a frustrating day or a bad week, these disorders color a victim's entire psychic life and can cause devastating changes in behavior and severe physical symptoms.

Major Depression

Signs and Symptoms

Major depression (discussed briefly in Chapters 3 and 4) is the most common of all mental illnesses. Between 10 and 20 percent of Americans will experience an episode at some time during their lives. As many as 2 percent of the nation's adolescents and adults are suffering from a depressive disorder today.

While the average age at which depression begins is in the late twenties, it can strike anyone, including infants, children and the elderly. Women are affected twice as often as men.

Unlike schizophrenia, depression is an *episodic* illness (see Appendix A). It lasts from two weeks to as long as two years, then disappears, leaving patients quite healthy, until it returns. Approximately 30 percent of those who experience one major depression never have to face another. The median number of episodes during a lifetime, however, is four.

The hallmarks of major depression include persistent *low mood*. The patient often complains of feeling sad, low or blue. In addition, he or she may look downcast, be easily moved to tears, speak quietly or hardly speak at all.

This low mood is almost always accompanied by a *loss of interest or pleasure in activities*. Things that used to bring the depressed person pleasure—whether food, sex, social events or work—no longer do.

One reason that activities lose their attraction is that patients frequently suffer *decreased physical and mental energy*. Their limbs may feel weighted down. The smallest task can seem insurmountable. People around the depressed person may notice that he or she moves sluggishly and seems slow to respond to questions or requests.

Difficulty with concentration and memory is not uncommon. Patients may complain, for example, that they cannot keep their attention focused on the newspaper or that they forget names, numbers and appointments. They may seem distractible or even disoriented.

The vast majority of patients will also experience *decreased appetite and weight loss*. Some patients, with less typical forms of depression, eat more and gain weight.

Disturbed sleep occurs in approximately 75 percent of patients. A small percentage sleep too much, but the vast majority of depressed people sleep too little. The most common problem is called *early morning awakening*: patients wake at 4 A.M. or 5 A.M. and cannot fall back to sleep. Others find it impossible to get to sleep to begin with and lie awake for hours worrying about the events of the day. Patients sometimes report being repeatedly roused by nightmares.

Bodily symptoms are common. Any part of the body may be involved. Headache, muscle cramps, back pain, blurred vision, constipation, indigestion and dry mouth are all frequent complaints.

Anxiety symptoms, including shortness of breath, feelings of inner restlessness, a sense of impending doom, "butterflies in the stomach," sweating and heart palpitations, can occur.

The patient's *self-esteem may plummet*. He or she may feel helpless, worthless or sinful.

The reasoning processes of some depressed individuals become so disordered that they may develop *delusions*. A depressed person may become convinced, for example, that he or she is personally responsible for all the crime in the world. *Hallucinations* can also occur.

Finally, depressed patients often brood over death and may struggle with recurrent *thoughts of suicide*.

Depression and Suicide

Suicide is the tenth leading cause of death in the United States. The rate among those aged fifteen to twenty-four has doubled over the past three decades, making suicide the second leading cause of death in young people.

The vast majority of suicides are due to major depression. As many as 15 percent of severely depressed people take their own lives.

The following, in a depressed patient, are signs of an increased risk of suicide:

1. Thoughts or talk of suicide
2. Hopelessness
3. Youth or old age [Suicide risk generally increases with age, but is particularly worrisome in adolescents, young adults and the elderly.]
4. A past history of a suicide attempt
5. A recent loss, such as the death of a spouse
6. An expressed belief that "reunion" with a loved one who has passed away may be possible
7. Isolation (including being single, separated, divorced or widowed), unemployment or an urban living environment
8. Medical illness, especially that involving chronic pain or a terminal diagnosis

Finally, one of the most dangerous periods for suicide in a severely depressed and suicidal person occurs when his or her condition responds partially to treatment and he or she is discharged from the hospital prematurely. At this point the depressed person may have just enough energy to carry out a plan for suicide and may not yet have enough optimism to reject the idea.

How Depression Varies With Age

Although the features of depression are similar in children, adolescents and adults, there are some differences.

In children, bodily symptoms and anxiety symptoms are particularly frequent. Auditory hallucinations, in which a single voice speaks to the child, are also common.

Depressed adolescents may show their distress by sulking, neglecting their personal appearance and withdrawing from the family. They may speak of feeling misunderstood by everyone around them. Moreover, they may become truant from school, break the law or begin using alcohol and drugs.

When depression occurs in the elderly, cognitive deficits such as memory loss, disorientation and confusion often predominate.

Bipolar Disorder

In bipolar disorder (once known as *manic-depressive illness*), the patient experiences periods of depression and its mirror image, called *mania* (discussed in Chapters 1 and 3). These depressive and manic episodes may follow directly on the heels of one another or may be separated by short or long intervals of normal mood.

Mania strikes one in every hundred people during their lifetimes. Men and women are at equal risk. Without ongoing treatment, as many as 75 percent of those who suffer one episode will have to face another.

The average age at which mania occurs is in the early twenties, but it affects people much later in life as well.

The following excerpt, taken from a classic case history written by psychiatrist Jacob Kasanin (1897–1946), captures some of the manic symptoms of a bipolar twenty-year-old laborer:

> Two weeks before admission the co-workers in the factory noticed that the patient began to talk a great deal and that he began to sing very loudly. Quite suddenly he declared that he was going on the stage or else would join a professional baseball team. The same behavior was observed at home. He sent a telegram to a Boston baseball team which was at that time playing in the South, asking the manager for a position. He told his family that he was going to make a great deal of money and they should finance him for the trip. He slept very poorly and was very restless at night. . . .
> . . . When in church he felt that the holy images might be alive and that God was in communication with him. . . .

The patient said that he could see God if he closed his eyes. He could see God moving about, saw Him moving His fingers and saw His features. He saw God sitting on the throne, pointing His fingers and controlling the movement of the world. God never talked to him. At one time he saw God mold clay and blow the breath of life into it.

Whereas mood is low in depression, in mania it is *elevated, irritable* or *hostile*. Mood may shift rapidly, swinging from elation, for example, to anger. The mood disturbance, together with the associated symptoms of mania, typically wreak havoc with the individual's job, social responsibilities or personal relationships.

One of the most frequent associated symptoms is *inflated self-esteem*. This can range from unwarranted self-confidence to true grandiosity. A manic person can even become *delusional,* believing that he or she is absolutely infallible or has famous friends that ensure success. He or she may attempt to market a frivolous new invention, make high-risk investments or suddenly change careers. As in Kasanin's patient, delusions can be extreme, such as having a special relationship to God. *Hallucinations* can also occur, often adding to the manic person's conviction that he or she is possessed of special powers.

When delusions and hallucinations are consistent with the patient's elevated mood, and with his or her having unusual powers, they are termed *mood congruent*. When they are frightening to the person (as in Oliver's case, described in Chapter 1), they are termed *mood incongruent*.

In mania, there is almost always a *decreased need for sleep*. Unlike depressed patients, manic patients may not be tired even after a series of sleepless nights. Patients typically, in fact, feel energized and *increase their activities*. Some work or study more, but others participate in dangerous pleasure seeking, such as sexual indiscretions or reckless driving. The behaviors can be bizarre, such as dressing in strange garb or preaching the word of God to passersby.

Not surprisingly, people suffering with mania are often *distractible*. Their attention wanders. A manic person, for example, may find it impossible to concentrate on a conversation when background noise is present.

Manic speech tends to be loud, rapid and difficult to understand. If the person's mood is elevated, his or her speech may be full of jokes and rhymes. If the person's predominant mood is irritable or hostile, he or she may sound angry or threatening. Anton Chekhov, the great Russian physician and writer, offered this description of a patient who seems to have been suffering with the *pressured speech* of mania:

> Soon, however, the urge to speak dominates all other considerations, and he unleashes his feelings, talking heatedly and passionately. His speech is disorganized, feverish, broken and not always intelligible, as in a delirium—but something exceptionally fine is nevertheless perceptible in his words and voice. . . . His mad harangue is hard to reproduce on paper. He talks about human vilainy, about violence crushing truth, about the splendid life there will be on earth in time, about window bars, reminding him every minute of the denseness and cruelty of the violators. It is a disorderly, disconnected potpourri put together out of the old refrains.

This kind of *flight of ideas*, in which patients chaotically rush from one thought to another, is common. Sometimes the rapid-fire thoughts remain unspoken, like ellipses between words. One manic patient, for example, gave his reason for buying a record album of Beethoven's music as, "I saw a man in the store with a cup of coffee." Only later did he explain the connection by quickly recapping his silent train of thought: "Coffee came from South America. Many Nazis went to South America after World War II. Nazis were from Germany. Beethoven was also from Germany."

Although the underlying suffering of those with mania is disguised by elevated mood and increased activity, patients who recover often describe the experience as a terrifying loss of control. They may reject help from others initially, but be more responsive to repeated demonstrations of concern.

Seasonal Affective Disorder

In some patients, major depression occurs at the same time each year, most often in November, at the leading edge of winter. In contrast to the typical depressive symptoms, these winter depressions tend to include *increased sleep, increased appetite* and *a craving for carbohydrates*.

Summer depressions also occur, usually with the more common symptoms of decreased sleep, decreased appetite and weight loss.

Between depressions, patients with seasonal affective disorder may experience mild or severe manic symptoms.

The notion that illness might be triggered at certain times of the year is far from new. Hippocrates himself believed that "it is chiefly the changes of seasons which produce diseases." Aristotle wrote that "cold beyond due measure . . . produces groundless despondency; hence suicide by hanging occurs."

Recurrent winter depressions are of particular interest to clinicians, because research seems to show that a decrease in the amount of sunlight reaching the retina (located at the back of the eye) causes them. Patients with this pattern of affective illness often improve when they are exposed each day to artificial bright lights, a relatively new and very exciting treatment called *phototherapy*.

Dysthymia and Cyclothymia

When groups of symptoms similar to those of depression and bipolar disorder are somewhat less intense, they are given different names. Patients who suffer from chronic low-level depression are diagnosed with dysthymia. Those who cycle regularly from mild depression to mild manic symptoms (*hypomania*) are diagnosed with cyclothymia.

Dysthymia and cyclothymia tend to begin gradually and to persist. For either condition to be diagnosed, in fact, symptoms must have been present almost continually for at least two years.

Like major depression and bipolar disorder, dysthymia and cyclothymia involve more than altered mood. Changes in physical and mental energy, self-esteem, concentration, sleep and appetite can also occur.

Because symptoms are less severe, patients with these two disorders often manage to continue functioning adequately at home and at work. They may even be particularly productive during the upward swing of cyclothymia.

Schizoaffective Disorder

In some patients, delusions and hallucinations are prominent during episodes of depression and mania, but also occur alone (without any dramatic mood symptoms) for weeks or more at a time.

These patients, who straddle the diagnostic boundaries between schizophrenia and mood disorders, are said to suffer with schizoaffective disorder.

A relatively small amount of data is available on those patients diagnosed with schizoaffective disorder. They seem to have chronic, rather than episodic, symptoms. Their chances for recovery are probably better than the chances of patients diagnosed with schizophrenia but not as good as those of patients with a pure mood disorder.

Many psychiatrists wonder whether schizoaffective disorder is really a separate psychiatric illness or just a variation of either schizophrenia, major depression or bipolar disorder. More research will be required to determine its diagnostic validity.

Are Mood Disorders Inherited?

A great deal of evidence has accumulated suggesting that mood disorders (especially bipolar disorder) are partly genetic. Much of the data comes from observations that the more closely two people are related, the less likely it is that a mood disorder will occur in just one of them. In fraternal twins, for example, when one twin has bipolar disorder, there is a 23 percent chance the other twin will develop it, too. But when the twins are identical, the likelihood of both being affected rises to 68 percent.

While bipolar disorder affects 1 to 2 percent of the general population, first-degree relatives of those with the disorder have a 10 to 25 percent risk of developing it.

Children with one parent suffering from bipolar disorder have a 25 percent chance of experiencing a serious mood disorder. If both parents are affected, the risk rises to 75 percent.

Cyclothymia and dysthymia also seem to occur more frequently in families that include close relatives with serious mood disorders.

Mood Disorders and the Brain

There is no shortage of theories linking major depression and bipolar disorder to brain chemistry. Researchers have known for a long time that patients with depression or bipolar disorder have alterations in the activity of the *biogenic amine family* of neurotransmitters, which includes norepinephrine, serotonin and dopamine.

Moreover, we know that the hypothalamus and pituitary glands, parts of the brain which regulate the secretion of many hormones, react differently in depressed patients. A hormone called cortisol, for example, ends up being produced in increased amounts, while the production of growth hormone and thyroid-stimulating hormone is suppressed.

We also have the example of *organic mood disorders*, in which symptoms nearly identical to those of major depression and mania have been caused by brain tumors, strokes or subtle seizures.

What we don't know is precisely how all these observations might be related or how they can result in the dramatic symptoms of affective illness. Some (as Freud himself initially did) argue that this gap in our knowledge will eventually yield to genetic, endocrinologic and neurologic research—that, ultimately, depression and mania will be translated into the language of hormones, chromosomes and neurotransmitters. Others, like myself, believe that, while neuroanatomy and neuropharmacology continue to harbor essential secrets, a complete understanding of mental disorders will always require uncovering the developmental and emotional issues of the individuals who suffer with them.

Medicines for Mood Disorders

Psychiatrists now have at hand a wide variety of medicines that are effective in treating the symptoms of major depression and bipolar disorder. These are extremely important adjuncts to psychotherapy in cases of moderate to severe affective disorder.

Because different medicines have different neurochemical effects and side effects, it can take some trial and error to settle on the best medicine (or combination of medicines) for a particular individual. Nonetheless, the vast majority of people treated for serious mood disorders eventually obtain significant, often quite dramatic, relief.

I say *eventually* because antidepressant and mood-stabilizing medications can take several weeks or even a few months to work. Scientists theorize that this delay in clinical improvement may exist because these medicines seem to exert their effects, in part, by slowly changing the number of receptors for various neurotransmitters, gradually modulating the "volume" of chemical communication between neurons.

Tricyclic Antidepressants

The tricyclic antidepressants were first introduced in 1957, with the drug imipramine. Others, including amitriptyline, desipramine and nortriptyline, followed (see Table 11–1). They are called *tricyclics* because of the three carbon rings that form the backbone of their chemical structures. Each acts as a *reuptake inhibitor* (see Chapter 9) of norepinephrine, serotonin or both, interfering with the normal reabsorption of these neurotransmitters into the cells that have just released them. Left to linger longer in the synaptic space around target neurons, these chemical messengers can continue to exert their effects.

This loitering of neurotransmitters in the synaptic space also seems to bring about the longer-term structural changes noted above. Because the amount of serotonin or norepinephrine in the synaptic space is greater, target cells effectively block their "ears" by reducing the number of their receptors for these chemicals.

Approximately 70 percent of patients treated with tricyclic antidepressants experience significant relief of depressive symptoms, usually within four to six weeks.

Like all psychoactive drugs, the tricyclics have side effects. These include sedation, low blood pressure (especially a fall in blood pressure upon standing) and anticholinergic effects (increased heart rate, constipation, blurred vision and dry mouth). For this reason, psychiatrists start these medicines slowly and then gradually increase dosages.

Because some of the tricyclics work best when their concentrations in the blood are kept within a fairly narrow range, frequent blood tests may be necessary.

Table 11–1. Tricyclic antidepressants

Generic name	Trade name(s)	Side effects		
		Sedation	Low blood pressure	Anticholinergic effects
Imipramine	Tofranil Presamine Janimine Imavate	Medium	More	Medium
Amitriptyline	Elavil Endep Amitril	More	More	More
Desipramine	Norpramin Pertofrane	Less	Less	Medium
Doxepin	Sinequan Adapin	More	Medium	More
Nortriptyline	Aventyl Pamelor	Less	Less	Medium
Protriptyline	Vivactil	Less	Medium	More
Trimipramine	Surmontil	More	Medium	More

Other Cyclic Antidepressants

Two four-ring antidepressants (i.e., quadricyclics)—maprotiline (Ludiomil) and amoxapine (Asendin)—were developed in the early 1980s. Each of these seems to be as effective as the tricyclics in relieving depression, but carries with it troubling side effects that have limited its use. Maprotiline is associated with an increased risk of seizures at high dosages. Amoxapine carries with it a small risk of tardive dyskinesia, the sometimes permanent movement disorder more commonly linked to antipsychotic medication.

Serotonin Reuptake Inhibitors

A number of antidepressants preferentially or exclusively exert their effects by altering the activity of a chemical messenger called serotonin, rather than norepinephrine. These medicines are as effective as the tricyclics and cause fewer anticholinergic side effects. They can, however, cause their own side effects, including gastrointestinal symptoms and sexual dysfunction.

One of these medicines, fluoxetine (Prozac), has been in the public eye since its approval in 1987 by the U.S. Food and Drug Administration (FDA). It has been lauded for its relative lack of side effects and has become the antidepressant most widely prescribed by psychiatrists in the United States. But it has also sparked lawsuits by a number of patients who allege that it caused them to behave violently toward themselves or others. An FDA panel has found no scientific basis for these claims.

Three other antidepressants that affect the serotonergic system are paroxetine (Paxil), sertraline (Zoloft) and trazodone (Desyrel). Trazodone tends to cause significant sedation and low blood pressure and is now mainly used to treat insomnia.

A fourth medication, called bupropion (Wellbutrin), which may work in part through the serotonergic system, carries an increased risk of seizures, particularly in those patients predisposed to them.

Monoamine Oxidase Inhibitors

If a tricyclic antidepressant or serotonin reuptake inhibitor fails to relieve the symptoms of depression, a monoamine oxidase inhibitor (MAOI) may be tried.

Monoamine oxidase is a normal enzyme in the body that breaks down neurotransmitters which routinely leak from storage depots in neurons. When the enzyme is inhibited (blocked), more neurotransmitter molecules are available to communicate with target neurons.

Three MAOIs—tranylcypromine (Parnate), phenelzine (Nardil) and isocarboxazid (Marplan)—are marketed in the United States. Although each can be used in any depressed patient, these medicines are thought to be particularly helpful to patients whose depressions include extreme anxiety, social phobias, sensitivity to being rejected, increased appetite and increased sleep.

MAOIs generally cause fewer anticholinergic side effects than do the tricyclic antidepressants, but they require a special diet. The reason for the dietary restrictions is that some foods (including cheeses, beer and red wine) contain an amino acid called *tyramine*, which can increase blood pressure. Normally, tyramine is broken down by monoamine oxidase. When this enzyme is inhibited, however, tyramine can accumulate to dangerous levels, potentially causing a life-threatening *hypertensive crisis*.

Certain medications (including other antidepressants), if taken in conjunction with MAOIs, can also bring about dangerous side effects. Therefore, use of MAOIs requires especially careful monitoring by a psychiatrist.

Lithium

Lithium, a naturally occurring salt, was first used in 1949 by an Australian psychiatrist named John Cade. Cade administered the salt to a man who had been in a terribly agitated state for five years. Within a few weeks, the patient's mood returned to normal.

Lithium carbonate (Eskalith, Lithobid, Lithotabs, etc.) has since proven to be a remarkably effective treatment for acute episodes of both mania and depression and has become the medicine upon which psychiatrists most frequently rely to prevent recurrences of either mood disorder.

No one understands exactly how lithium works. Its effectiveness highlights the fact that we really know very little about the physical basis of mood disorders. Like so many of our treatments aimed at the brain, lithium works, but we don't know why.

Common side effects of lithium treatment include mild hand tremor, weight gain, nausea, diarrhea, increased thirst and increased urination. Of much more concern are the signs of lithium toxicity, including confusion, lack of coordination and severe tremulousness.

Because of the potential dangers of toxicity, lithium's concentration in the blood must be monitored with frequent blood tests. Blood tests are also used to make sure that thyroid function and kidney function, either of which can be disturbed by lithium, remain normal.

Antiseizure Medications

At least two medicines normally used to treat patients with epilepsy—carbamazepine (Tegretol) and valproic acid (Depakene)—are also effective in controlling mood disorders in some patients. This has led to speculation that these disorders might be caused, in part, by very subtle seizures in the brain. We know, after all, that temporal lobe epilepsy can itself mimic the signs and symptoms of major depression (see Chapter 9).

The theory is complicated, however, by the fact that antiseizure medicines not only alter the brain's electrical activity but also affect its neurotransmitter systems.

Side effects of these two medicines include diarrhea, constipation, incoordination and, rarely, blood or liver disorders. Blood tests are required prior to, and during, treatment.

Combination Drug Treatment

Frequently, psychiatrists prescribe a combination of medications to optimize results. Lithium, for example, can enhance the effectiveness of some antidepressants. Two antidepressants used together (always under a psychiatrist's close supervision) sometimes work far better than either alone. Treatment of the psychotic symptoms of mania or depression may require addition of a neuroleptic (see Chapter 10). Antianxiety medications (see Chapter 12) can help to reduce a patient's irritability. Insomnia often calls for a sleep medicine.

What all of this means is that there is not only a good deal of science but also a fair measure of clinical artistry involved in the pharmacologic management of psychiatric illness. Patients can be assured that other creative medication strategies can be tried, even when the first, second and third fail to relieve these patients' symptoms.

Electroconvulsive Therapy

Electroconvulsive therapy (ECT) is psychiatry's most controversial treatment. It involves passing a pulse of electricity through a patient's brain in order to cause a seizure. By mechanisms as mysterious as those underlying the benefits of mood-stabilizing medications, these seizures can lead to dramatic relief of major depression and mania.

The bad reputation that ECT has acquired is largely a legacy of its youth. After being discovered by the Italian psychiatrists Ugo Cerletti and Lucio Bini more than five decades ago, hospitals tended to use it indiscriminately and without anesthesia. In these circumstances miraculous recoveries were documented, but the results were often temporary and the treatment dangerous, at times causing broken bones, heart attacks and brain damage.

Hollywood, as in *One Flew Over the Cuckoo's Nest,* did its part by portraying ECT as a way of punishing free thinkers and controlling their minds.

Today's technically refined ECT is making something of a comeback. Less electrical current is used, and the duration of the pulse is limited to approximately two seconds. The patient is given anesthesia, which puts him or her to sleep and completely relaxes his or her muscles. This means that the seizure activity that occurs in the brain can't lead to generalized body convulsions. The procedure takes about twenty minutes start to finish. It is usually repeated six to twelve times, over several weeks, until symptoms are relieved.

Because it continues to be stigmatized and because it requires anesthesia, ECT is still generally reserved for hospitalized patients whose depressions have failed to respond to medications. Some studies show that as many as 90 percent of these patients improve with ECT. It is also an option when patients are suffering especially troubling symptoms, such as near-starvation, severe psychosis or persistent thoughts of suicide, that demand prompt relief.

The side effects of ECT include memory loss; 40 percent of patients report a spotty loss of new and old memories. This is generally a temporary problem (weeks to months), but some patients have reported more lasting amnesia, usually for events that occurred around the time of treatment.

Other side effects include nausea, headache, muscle ache and the infrequent, but potentially serious, problems associated with anesthesia.

Remembering Oliver and Maria

Nowhere in this chapter can the reader find the entirety of Oliver's and Maria's experiences with mental illness (see Chapters 1 and 4). True, they fit the descriptions of mania and major depression, respectively. Thankfully, matching them with those diagnoses helped to direct me to effective medications. The diagnostic labels even allowed me some insight into possible brain abnormalities underlying their symptoms and predicted the episodic course of their illnesses. None of this, however, was a substitute for knowing each of them as a person and acknowledging that the pain each felt was unique, a product of his or her singular life experience. Oliver's kidnapped family members and Maria's burning feet weren't just an anonymous delusion or hallucination—inert items on a checklist. They were like fingerprints of their suffering.

Attention to the details of these fingerprints is an essential component of the treatment of mental disorders and emotional distress. Simply medicating the disorder and not healing the person behind it would be akin to repairing a car's transmission, never addressing the fact that the driver feels compelled to race along highways in first gear.

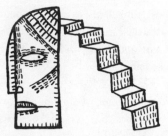

12

Anxiety Disorders

The Schoolmaster

In "The Schoolmaster," Emil Kraepelin describes a patient who suffers with both hypochondriasis and a debilitating anxiety disorder:

The patient is quite collected, clear, and well-ordered in his statements. He says that one of his sisters suffers in the same way as himself. He traces the beginning of his illness back to about eleven years ago. Being a clever lad, he became a schoolmaster, and had to do a great deal of mental work to qualify. Gradually he began to fear that he had a serious disease, and was going to die of heart apoplexy. All the assurances and examinations of his doctor could not convince him. For this reason he suddenly left his appointment and went home one day, seven years ago, being afraid that he would die shortly. After this he consulted every possible doctor, and took long holidays repeatedly, always recovering a little, but invariably finding that his fears returned speedily. These were gradually reinforced by the fear of gatherings of people. He was also unable to cross large squares or go through wide streets by himself. He avoided using the railway for fear of collisions and derailments, and he would not travel in a boat lest it might capsize. He was seized with apprehension on bridges and when skating, and at last the apprehension of apprehension itself caused palpitations and oppression on all sorts of occasions. . . . On the way here, when he had finally made up his mind to place himself in our hands, he trembled with deadly fear.

The patient describes himself as a chicken-hearted fellow, who, in spite of good mental ability, has always been afraid of all sorts of diseases—consumption, heart apoplexy, and the like. He knows that these anxieties are morbid, yet cannot free himself from them. This apprehensiveness came out in a very marked way while he was under observation in the hospital. He worried about every remedy, whether it was baths, packs, or medicine, being afraid it would be too strong for him, and have a weakening effect. He always wished to have a warder within call in case he got agitated. The sight of other patients disturbed him greatly, and when he went for a walk in the garden with the door shut he was tormented by the fear of not being able to get out of it in case anything happened. At last he would hardly venture in front of the house, and always had to have the door open behind him so that he could take refuge indoors in case of necessity. He begged to have a little bottle of "blue electricity" that he had brought with him to give him confidence. Sometimes he was seized with violent palpitation of the heart while he was sitting down. . . . It struck him that his look had got very gloomy, and he thought it was the beginning of a mental disturbance which would certainly seize upon him while he was here.

A Group of Illnesses

Anxiety disorders, which include panic disorder, phobias, obsessive-compulsive disorder, and posttraumatic stress disorder, all cause high, often debilitating, levels of anxiety or fear. In attempting to avoid the discomfort, many patients dramatically alter their personal habits, social interactions or work activities.

In some cases, as with phobias, the source of the patient's anxiety is clear; fear of heights and of crowds are two examples. But in other cases, as with panic attacks, absolute terror can strike unpredictably, when a patient is simply reading a book or taking a leisurely walk.

Panic Disorder

Panic disorder, which affects millions of Americans, is a sudden, overwhelming terror that seems to come out of the blue. As in the schoolmaster's case, the fear is accompanied by symptoms such as shortness of breath, sweating, feelings of numbness or tingling, a choking sensation, heart palpitations and trembling. Some patients fear they are going out of their minds or have lost all touch with reality. They may feel that they are about to do something crazy and uncontrollable or that they are about to die.

It is not unusual for someone suffering a panic attack to rush to an emergency room, believing he or she is having a heart attack. As many as one-third of those who arrive at emergency rooms complaining of chest pain, in fact, are actually suffering from panic disorder.

Panic disorder usually begins in a person's late twenties. It affects women more often than men, but both sexes are vulnerable to it.

Some individuals never experience a second attack, but, much more frequently, the attacks occur again and again, often for years.

Unfortunately, few of those who experience panic attacks understand from the outset that their fear is the result of a known and treatable illness. They begin to avoid those situations in which their attacks happen, by chance, to have occurred. Possibly in this way, panic disorder often comes to be coupled with *agoraphobia,* a fear of being in an area (such as a crowded street) where getting away or getting help in case of emergency would be difficult. Patients may dramatically curtail their lifestyles—never driving or rarely leaving the house. They may try to self-medicate their symptoms with alcohol or drugs, an ill-advised strategy which ultimately only increases anxiety.

It is essential that potential bodily causes of "panic" be excluded by a full medical history and physical examination. Thyroid disease, drug use (or withdrawal) and certain tumors can cause symptoms that are nearly indistinguishable from those of pure panic disorder.

Phobias

Winston could hear the blood singing in his ears. He had the feeling of sitting in utter loneliness. He was in the middle of a great empty plain, a flat desert drenched with sunlight, across which all sounds came to him out of immense distances. Yet the cage with the rats was not two meters away from him. They were enormous rats. They were at the age when a rat's muzzle grows blunt and fierce and his fur brown instead of gray.... There was an outburst of squeals from the cage. It seemed to reach Winston from far away. The rats were fighting; they were trying to get at each other through the partition. He heard also a deep groan of despair. That, too, seemed to come from out-side himself. . . . Suddenly the foul musty odor of the brutes struck his nostrils. There was a violent convulsion of nausea inside him, and he almost lost consciousness. Everything had gone black. For an instant he was insane, a screaming animal.

This gripping description of a fictional character's fear of rats (called a *simple phobia*) was written by novelist George Orwell, in his book *1984*. In phobias the source of fear and anxiety is a specific object or situation well known to the patient. Frederick the Great, for example, was afraid of water and wouldn't bathe. Edgar Allan Poe was terrified of confining spaces, a fear he described in stories like "The Premature Burial."

Between 3 and 5 percent of the population suffer from phobias, which tend to begin in late childhood. They are twice as common in women as in men.

Faced with the dreaded object or situation, a phobic individual can become immediately terrified and may experience all the symptoms of panic, including palpitations, sweating, dizziness, shortness of breath and an intense desire to flee. Some patients, like Orwell's fictional character Winston, also report a sense of being outside their bodies or feeling strangely removed and disconnected from their immediate surroundings. Having endured this suffering, people with phobias may go to extreme lengths to avoid another encounter with that which they fear, sometimes leading to severe problems in coping with their work environments or social relationships.

For diagnostic purposes, phobias are divided into three categories: simple phobia, agoraphobia (discussed earlier in this chapter) and *social phobia*.

Simple phobias are excessive fears of specific objects—like Winston's fear of rats. Other examples are the fear of closed spaces (*claustrophobia*) and of heights (*acrophobia*).

Agoraphobia, which is usually coupled with panic attack, is the fear of being alone in public places from which escape might be difficult or help hard to find in case of emergency. The emergencies people with agoraphobia tend to dread are incapacitating or embarrassing ones, such as fainting, having a heart attack, vomiting, or losing bowel or bladder control. People suffering with agoraphobia most often attempt to avoid crowded or isolated places, including congested bridges, back roads, department stores or street rallies. Pierre Janet, a French psychiatrist and contemporary of Freud, described a young man suffering from the disorder:

> He was about 25 years old when there started what he himself called "the trouble with spaces." He was crossing the Place de la Concorde (alone, it should be noted) when he felt a strange sensation of dread. His breathing became rapid and he felt as if he were suffocating; his heart was beating violently, and his legs were limp as if half paralyzed. He could go neither forwards nor backwards, and he had to exert a tremendous effort, bathed in sweat, to reach the other side of the square. From the time of that first episode on, he took a great dislike to the Place de la Concorde and decided that he would not risk going there again alone. However, a short while after, the same sensation of anxiety recurred on the Invalides Bridge, and then in a street, which though it was narrow, seemed long and was quite steep.
>
> . . . The anxiety he would experience whenever he had to venture out into a place that was at all open was so severe that it became impossible for him to control it, and he was no longer able to cross any square. Some dozen years ago he had had to escort a young girl to her house. As long as he was with her everything was all right, but when she had left him, he was unable to go back home. Five hours later, noticing that although it was getting dark and was raining, he had not yet returned, his wife became alarmed and went out in search of him. She found him ashen and shivering with cold on the edge of the Place des Invalides, which he had been completely unable to cross.

Social phobia, which is less common than simple phobia or agoraphobia, is the irrational fear and avoidance of being watched or humiliated by others in particular situations. The situations that inspire fear can be as seemingly routine as swallowing, so that patients choke on food when trying to eat in public. Others find it impossible to use public lavatories or to speak in front of more than one person.

Obsessive-Compulsive Disorder

Patients suffering with obsessive-compulsive disorder (OCD) are at the mercy of disturbing, repetitive thoughts, images or ideas that they cannot "get out of [their] minds."

The individual affected may recognize these *obsessions* as irrational and attempt to banish them, but usually without much success. A patient may, for example, be preoccupied with the fear of accidently harming others. He or she may worry constantly over being physically or spiritually unclean. Philosophical or religious questions may occupy the person ceaselessly and never be resolved.

Compulsions are the rituals that patients perform to neutralize the anxiety caused by obsessions. An individual who obsesses over inadvertently harming his family, for example, may feel compelled to touch a light switch a dozen times in order to make certain the house will not catch fire. A patient obsessed with germs may feel compelled to wash up again and again (perhaps for hours) before work or to say a special prayer to be sure no disease will be carried to co-workers. The most common compulsions involve hand washing, counting, checking and touching.

One of Sigmund Freud's now-famous case histories describes a young man suffering with OCD (then termed "obsessional neurosis"). The patient's compulsive behavior is fueled by his obsessional fear that harm might befall a woman he admires:

> . . . as they were sitting together during a thunderstorm, he was obsessed, he could not tell why, with the *necessity for counting* up to forty or fifty between each flash of lightning and its accompanying thunderclap. On the day of her departure he knocked his foot against a stone lying in the road, and was *obliged* to put it out of the way by the side of the road, because the idea struck him that her carriage would be driving along the same road in a few hours' time and might come to grief against this stone. But a few minutes later it occurred to him that this was absurd, and he was *obliged* to go back and replace the stone in its original position in the middle of the road.

OCD most often begins in late childhood or early adolescence. It is equally common in men and women.

Posttraumatic Stress Disorder

Posttraumatic stress disorder (PTSD) can strike anyone who survives a severe physical or mental trauma. The disorder has gained notoriety from the frequency with which it afflicts war veterans, but a much wider population, including children, are at risk. This population includes, for example, people who have been beaten, raped, tortured or witness to gruesome accidents, catastrophes or natural disasters.

Symptoms of PTSD can appear soon after the trauma or be delayed months or even years. But, eventually, people with the disorder begin to reexperience the traumatic event or the anxiety associated with it. The most dramatic symptoms are the distressing recollections, nightmares or daytime *flashbacks* in which the trauma is "replayed." Nightmares can be so severe that patients wake from sleep screaming. Flashbacks can include a *dissociative state* in which victims actually lose touch with reality. A Vietnam veteran who has a flashback while walking through a familiar neighborhood, for example, might be convinced he is in hostile territory and frantically seek cover from the enemy.

Other symptoms include a kind of emotional anesthesia called *psychic numbing*, which leaves patients disinterested in the world around them. They may withdraw from family and friends, leaving themselves increasingly isolated.

Patients often try particularly hard to avoid situations that remind them of their traumas. Even minor similarities can trigger symptoms. Someone who has been severely assaulted by a policeman, for example, may avoid watching television, lest a similar situation be depicted. Someone who watched a friend drown may attempt to avoid seeing any body of water. This avoidance behavior can become so consuming that patients are nearly housebound.

Some victims of PTSD report being extremely "touchy," easily startled or easily moved to anger and violence. They can experience all the symptoms of panic disorder.

PTSD also leaves people at risk for depression (see Chapter 11). Low mood, insomnia, difficulty concentrating, feelings of guilt and bodily aches and pains are all common complaints.

In some cases, particularly when symptoms develop soon after a single traumatic event, PTSD stops spontaneously within six months. In many cases, however, the disorder continues for years.

Are Anxiety Disorders Inherited?

It is very unclear to what extent, if any, genetic inheritance plays a role in anxiety disorders. Researchers have tried to determine whether personal characteristics like shyness, nervousness and fearfulness run in families. The data only hint at a possible genetic factor. Studies show, for example, that if one identical twin is particularly fearful and tense, the other twin is likely to be fearful and tense, even if the two were raised separately.

Based on the information at hand, psychiatrists have not come to any firm conclusions about anxiety disorders being inherited.

Anxiety Disorders and the Brain

The evidence linking anxiety disorders to bodily abnormalities began with research on panic disorder. As early as the 1940s, Harvard scientists had noted that panic sufferers who complained of worsening symptoms with exercise had unusually high levels of lactate—a normal body chemical produced by muscular exertion—in their blood. Other investigators, curious to see whether lactate might be the chemical key to panic, injected it into the bloodstreams of patients who had suffered with the disorder. Their symptoms quickly returned.

Later research implicated certain neurotransmitters. People with anxiety disorders were found to have increased activity of the excitatory catecholamine neurotransmitters (which include epinephrine) and decreased activity of an inhibitory neurotransmitter called gamma-aminobutyric acid (GABA).

Recently, imaging studies of the brains of panic-prone individuals have been conducted using positron-emission tomography (PET; see Chapter 9). These studies show abnormal patterns of blood flow and metabolism in an area of the brain called the *parahippocampal gyrus*, known to be associated with the expression of emotion and fear. PET scanning has also revealed abnormal metabolism in the *caudate nucleus* of patients with OCD. The caudate nucleus is a part of the brain which, in animals, controls instinctive and repetitive behaviors, like grooming.

As was the case in major depression (see Chapter 11), hormonal abnormalities have also been implicated in anxiety disorders. A percentage of victims release abnormal levels of certain hormones from the thyroid, hypothalamus and adrenal glands.

Medicines for Anxiety Disorders

Several kinds of medication, used in conjunction with psychotherapy or behavior therapy, are effective in relieving the symptoms of anxiety disorders. These medications differ dramatically in chemical structure and have very different effects on the brain. As was the case in treating depression and mania, these biological remedies often work quite well, but we can't explain exactly why.

Many of the medicines that are useful in treating anxiety disorders, in fact, are also useful in treating mood disorders, leading scientists to wonder about a biological link between the two.

The *tricyclic antidepressants* and *monoamine oxidase inhibitors* (see Chapter 11), for example, have been particularly helpful in reducing symptoms of panic disorder, posttraumatic stress disorder and social phobia.

OCD responds best to a tricyclic antidepressant called clomipramine (Anafranil). Clomipramine seems to affect the serotonergic system, leading to speculation that serotonin reuptake inhibitors (see Chapter 11), such as fluoxetine (Prozac), paroxetine (Paxil) and sertraline (Zoloft), might also be of use.

Other medications include *beta-blockers* like propranolol (Inderal) and atenolol (Tenormin). Beta-blockers are normally prescribed for high blood pressure, but can reduce palpitations, sweating and trembling in patients with social phobia.

Anxiety disorders are often treated with benzodiazepine "tranquilizers," such as clonazepam (Klonopin), alprazolam (Xanax), diazepam (Valium), lorazepam (Ativan) and oxazepam (Serax). Treatment with these medications is complicated because patients prone to substance abuse may misuse them and because the medications increase the intoxicating effects of alcohol. Moreover, some of the benzodiazepines, if stopped abruptly or used sporadically, can actually increase agitation and even lead to symptoms of withdrawal, including seizures.

A relatively new antianxiety medicine, called buspirone (BuSpar), is sometimes effective in relieving anxiety without bringing the drowsiness and addictive potential of the benzodiazepines. Buspirone, however, takes up to four weeks to work and is, therefore, not useful as an immediate remedy for acute symptoms.

Each of the medicines discussed has its own side effects and should only be used after a full discussion of their risks and benefits with a physician.

Entrée to the Mind

Many of the best strategies for treating anxiety disorders (and other psychiatric conditions) involve medicines only peripherally or not at all. The success of various psychotherapies in alleviating symptoms of panic, phobias, OCD and PTSD testifies to the power of treatments aimed at the mind, rather than the brain. The third section of this book is dedicated to describing the ways in which psychiatrists think about the mind and to outlining the very effective strategies we have developed to heal it.

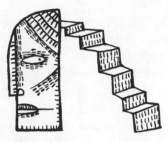

13

Personality Disorders

The "Psychopathic" Personality

Hervey Cleckley, a psychiatrist and the author of The Mask of Sanity, *wrote in the 1950s of a patient who, while outwardly quite congenial, seemed emotionally disabled in a way that resulted in painful consequences for himself and others. Cleckley diagnosed his patient, Tom, with psychopathic personality. Today, Tom's symptoms would fit with what we call antisocial personality disorder:*

This young man, 21 years of age, does not look at all like a criminal type or a shifty delinquent. . . .

Tom looks and is in robust physical health. His manner and appearance are pleasing. . . .

. . . [His] immediate problem was serious but not monumental. His family and legal authorities were in hope that if some psychiatric disorder could be discovered in him, he might escape a jail sentence for stealing. . . .

Evidence of his maladjustment became distinct in childhood. He appeared to be a reliable and manly fellow but could never be counted upon to keep at any task or to give a straight account of any situation. He was frequently truant from school. . . . Though he was generously provided for, he stole some of his father's chickens from time to time, selling them at stores downtown. Pieces of table silver would be missed. These were sometimes recovered from those to whom he had sold them for a pittance or swapped them for odds and ends which seemed to hold no particular interest or value for him. . . .

Often when truant from high school classes, Tom wandered more or less aimlessly, sometimes shooting at . . . chickens, setting fire to a rural privy around the outskirts of town, or perhaps loitering about a cigar store or a pool room, reading the comics, throwing rocks at squirrels in a park, perpetrating small thefts or swindles. . . .

He lied so plausibly and with such equanimity, devised such ingenious alibis or simply denied all responsibility with such convincing appearances of candor that for many years his real career was poorly estimated. . . .

Though he often fell in with groups or small gangs, he never for long identified himself with others in a common cause. . . .

Reliable information indicates that he has been arrested and imprisoned approximately fifty or sixty times. It is estimated that he would have been put in jails or police barracks for short or long periods of detention on approximately 150 other occasions if his family had not made good his small thefts and damages and paid fines for him. . . .

This young man apparently has never formed any substantial attachment for another person. Sexually he has been desultorily promiscuous under a wide variety of circumstances. A year or two earlier he married a girl who had achieved considerable local recognition as a prostitute and as one whose fee was moderate. He had previously shared her offerings during an evening (on a commercial basis) with friends or with brief acquaintances among whom he found himself. He soon left the bride and never showed any signs of shame or chagrin about the character of the woman he had espoused or of any responsibility toward her.

When Is a Personality a Disorder?

All of us know people who have qualities that are irritating or seem counterproductive. We develop catchphrases to describe these irksome personality traits: Paul *thinks he's God*; Heather's *afraid of her own shadow*; Max is *on another planet*; Kelly's *bad news*; John's *his own worst enemy*.

When an individual's personality traits remain rigid despite the fact that they interfere significantly with his or her happiness or ability to function in the world, psychiatrists label them as disorders. Tom's contempt for rules and lack of regard for the feelings of others, unchanged by consequences like repeated imprisonment, is one example.

This is a relatively new, controversial and rapidly evolving diagnostic arena. The implications of calling particular types of people *disordered* are tremendous. It raises concerns about whether psychiatry, by labeling odd or unruly people as sick, could become a homogenizing force in society. It also raises the question of whether people like Cleckley's patient are really responsible for what they do.

By current diagnostic standards, approximately 10 percent of the population fit one or another personality disorder. Overall, males are affected as often as females. The disorders are more common in lower socioeconomic classes and in disadvantaged communities.

In the descriptions that follow, you may identify characteristics of friends, relatives or yourself. Keep in mind that it is only when several personality symptoms cluster into an inflexible, harmful syndrome that a personality disorder is diagnosed.

Dramatic, Erratic Personalities

Antisocial Personality Disorder

Like Tom, people with *antisocial personality disorder* have a chronic disregard for the rights of others that is obvious from their irresponsible and, often, unlawful behavior. The disorder begins as *conduct disorder* in childhood or early adolescence (always by age fifteen) and continues into adulthood, only being diagnosed once the individual reaches eighteen years of age.

Early on, people with antisocial personality disorder seem to be at war with the world. They may lie frequently, steal, be truant from school, show cruelty to animals or to other people, engage in physical fights, destroy property and deliberately set fires. Later (after age fifteen), it often becomes obvious that the person is unable to keep a job, is overtly aggressive and reckless, fails to honor the law, has no regard for the truth and feels no remorse after hurting others.

Antisocial personality disorder is much more common in males than females. People with the disorder also tend to use illicit drugs and to be sexually active at a relatively early age.

Borderline Personality Disorder

One of my patients, then approaching age forty, had been admitted to psychiatric facilities hundreds of times. The typical scenario resulting in his admission was that one of his on-and-off, chaotic romances or friendships would falter and, in order to relieve his mounting feelings of anxiety and depression, he would drink heavily and then cut his forearms with a razor. Bloodied and inebriated, he would either call an emergency room for an ambulance or walk right in.

On the ward, he had acquired a reputation for testing the rules and fostering disputes between staff members about them. When he felt left out or slighted by any other patient or staff member, he was quick to threaten suicide, making it necessary for him to be observed around the clock. At the point when leaving the ward was discussed, his symptoms would worsen, and, on several occasions, he would make unsuccessful attempts on his life, preventing his discharge.

My patient suffered with *borderline personality disorder*, a condition marked by a fear of and inability to tolerate being alone. This fear leads to behaviors such as substance abuse, promiscuity and threats or actual episodes of self-destructiveness. Often the threats are designed to manipulate others. Relationships are typically intense and unstable, with the patient alternately overvaluing and devaluing their importance. Often, individuals with the disorder report chronic troubling feelings, with mood swings from rage to depression, emptiness or boredom.

Histrionic Personality Disorder

Emil Kraepelin described *histrionic personality disorder* in one of his classic case histories, an excerpt of which follows:

> With her growing expertness in illness, the emotional sympathies of the patient are more and more confined to the selfish furthering of her own wishes. She tries ruthlessly to extort the most careful attention from those around her ... The sacrifices made by others, more especially by her family, are regarded quite as a matter of course, and her occasional prodigality of thanks only serves to pave the way for new demands. To secure the sympathy of those around her, she has recourse to more and more forcible descriptions of her physical and

mental torments, histrionic exaggeration of her attacks, and the effective elucidation of her personal character. She calls herself the abandoned, the outcast, and in mysterious hints makes confession of horrible, delightful experiences and failings, which she will only confide to the discreet bosom of her very best friend, the doctor.

Like Kraepelin's patient, people with histrionic personality disorder are overly emotional and attention seeking. Because they use their appearance, style of communication and behavior to elicit and maintain the interest and approval of those around them, they often dress or behave seductively, flamboyantly or inappropriately. They crave novelty and excitement and are easily bored. Faced with situations in which they cannot be the focus of attention, they become uncomfortable and frustrated.

Histrionic individuals tend to overreact, being moved to tears, anger or obvious joy. To others, therefore, their emotions often seem unwarranted. Similarly, their speech may seem excessively impressionistic and lacking in detail. For example, when asked to describe his or her mother, such a person might not be able to expand beyond a brush stroke description like, "She was a wonderful person."

Other features of the disorder are a tendency to be overly trusting of others and suggestible and to "play hunches."

Narcissistic Personality Disorder

His brown, hardening body lived naturally through the half-fierce, half-lazy work of the bracing days. He knew women early, and since they spoiled him he became contemptuous of them, of young virgins because they were ignorant, of the others because they were hysterical about things which in his overwhelming self-absorption he took for granted.

But his heart was in a constant, turbulent riot. The most grotesque and fantastic conceits haunted him in his bed at night. A universe of ineffable gaudiness spun itself out in his brain while the clock ticked on the washstand and the moon soaked with wet light his tangled clothes upon the floor. Each night he added to the pattern of his fancies until drowsiness closed down upon some vivid scene with an oblivious embrace.

This description (and those that follow) of the fictional character Jay Gatsby was written by novelist F. Scott Fitzgerald. Gatsby illustrates many of the symptoms of *narcissistic personality disorder*, a condition marked primarily by a pervasive pattern of grandiosity, hypersensitivity to criticism and a lack of empathy.

People with this disorder tend to exaggerate their importance, talents and achievements. They feel unique and entitled, and expect to be seen and treated as "special." Yet their underlying self-esteem is most often fragile; when they fail to perform perfectly, they may be overly critical, or frankly ashamed, of themselves. They need to be admired and may be preoccupied with how well they are *doing* in the eyes of others and where they rank in a social, intellectual or physical hierarchy of their peers.

> "I'm going to make a big request of you today," he [Gatsby] said, pocketing his souvenirs with satisfaction, "so I thought you ought to know something about me. I didn't want you to think I was just some nobody."

They spend much mental energy fantasizing about unlimited success and power and are intensely envious of those they perceive as being more successful than they are. When they actually pursue large goals, it is often with joyless and extreme drive.

Narcissistic people tend to form friendships based on a sense that they can profit from them. Romantic partners are likely to be treated as objects selected to bolster the narcissist's self-esteem.

> There must have been moments even that afternoon when Daisy tumbled short of his dreams—not through her own fault, but because of the colossal vitality of his illusion. It had gone beyond her, beyond everything. He had thrown himself into it with a creative passion, adding to it all the time, decking it out with every bright feather that drifted his way.

Odd, Eccentric Personalities

Paranoid Personality Disorder

Individuals with *paranoid personality disorder* are intensely suspicious and mistrustful of others, without any justifiable reason. Because they see people as likely to exploit or harm them, they are reluctant to confide in family, friends or associates without being shown unusual demonstrations of loyalty or trustworthiness. They are often intensely jealous and, if disappointed or slighted, may be utterly unforgiving. They perceive the world as a hostile place.

A successful middle-aged businessman I treated, for example, was referred to me after he became intensely suspicious that his partners had it in mind to derail one of his banking deals. He described his view that acquaintances, colleagues and family members had been, over the course of decades, involved in various subtle intrigues against him— "playing games with him," he put it. He saw himself as a self-styled loner too complex for most people to understand. He had intentionally selected a single friend and confidant, from whom he had demanded and received a written promise of allegiance, signed by a drop of blood from each of them.

The defensiveness of paranoid individuals can lead them to be argumentative and quick to retaliate when they perceive any criticism or threat. They may seem overly serious, stubborn, hostile, insensitive or "cold."

Such people tend to shun group activities and show an excessive need to be self-sufficient. They are keenly aware of rank and may envy those in power while having contempt for those "below" them.

Even though difficulties with personal and occupational relationships are common, paranoid individuals often keep their ideas to themselves and continue to function adequately at work. They may even excel at projects that require analytic or strategic thinking.

During periods of unusual stress, however, people with paranoid personality disorder may become transiently psychotic.

It is important to note that the symptoms of this disorder can be mimicked by chronic abuse of amphetamines or cocaine.

Schizoid and Schizotypal Personality Disorders

The central feature of *schizoid personality disorder* is emotional and social detachment from others, with a lifelong pattern of isolation. Unlike paranoid individuals, people with this disorder rarely express strong emotions themselves and are indifferent to the feelings and opinions of others. They avoid close relationships, including sexual ones. Almost always, they favor solitary activities, which often include scientific or futuristic theories.

The following excerpt from the case history of a fifty-year-old retired policeman brings the symptoms to life:

> He prefers to be by himself, finds talk a waste of time, and feels awkward when other people try to initiate a relationship. . . . He is employed as a security guard, but is known by fellow workers as a "cold fish" and a "loner." They no longer even notice or tease him, especially since he never seemed to notice or care about their teasing anyway.
>
> John floats through life without relationships except for that with his dog, which he dearly loved. . . . He experienced the death of his parents without emotion, and feels no regret whatever at being completely out of contact with the rest of his family. He considers himself different from other people, and regards emotionality in others with bewilderment.

Schizotypal personality disorder also includes symptoms of social isolation and lack of emotional expression. Schizotypal individuals, however, tend to be more suspicious of others and to show more eccentricities in the way they look, think, speak and perceive the world around them. They are given, for example, to superstitions and to beliefs in magical kinds of communication, such as clairvoyance and a "sixth sense." They sometimes describe unusual perceptions, like sensing an "evil force" in a room or feeling "the presence" of a deceased loved one. They may speak abstractly or seem to wander off the topic being discussed.

A young woman I treated, for example, was admitted to the hospital ward after coming to the emergency room one night, without any money or a place to sleep, and expressing intense concerns about an approaching "day of judgment." She had been living in a religious commune but had left there after a deceased relative in a dream told her to. Part of her commitment to the religion (although not advocated by the commune elders) was eating only certain beans and oils. All other foods, she explained, were "poisonous" to the "spirit." She would occasionally talk about her life history and about her plans for the future, but almost always wandered into lengthy allusions to spiritual and mystical matters. She considered her family history "irrelevant." Although she asked for help in finding an interim place to live, she asserted convincingly that she was perfectly happy with her belief system, was not interested in therapy or medication, and wished only to prepare for Armageddon, looming perhaps a decade hence.

Schizoid and schizotypal personality disorders obviously have some symptoms—emotional constriction and social isolation, for example—in common with schizophrenia. The difference is that schizophrenia also includes an active phase of relatively long-lived and severe psychosis (e.g., hearing voices, seeing visions or having fixed and false beliefs).

Anxious, Fearful Personalities

Avoidant Personality Disorder

Leon attended college and did well for a while, then dropped out as his grades slipped. He remained very self-conscious and "terrified" of meeting strangers. He had trouble finding a job because he was unable to answer questions in interviews. He worked a few jobs for which only a written test was required . . . but refused . . . several promotions because he feared the social pressures.

Leon displays symptoms of *avoidant personality disorder*. People with this disorder are unusually timid and fearful, especially in situations in which people might reject or criticize them. They worry about saying "something stupid" or reacting inappropriately—for example, by crying or laughing at the wrong time—at parties or meetings. For this reason, they tend to avoid social and occupational gatherings in which they might be judged harshly by others. They are likely to refuse promotions or jobs that require them to attend many such functions. Because they are most comfortable with the routine they know, they exaggerate the risks or difficulties involved in doing anything different, such as meeting for dinner in a location they are unfamiliar with or traveling to a wedding in another city.

Unlike isolated and reclusive patients with schizoid personality disorder, patients with avoidant personality disorder actually yearn for interpersonal contact and are frustrated by the discomfort they experience in dealing with others.

Passive-Aggressive Personality Disorder

The symptoms of *passive-aggressive personality disorder* all revolve around the central theme that the person with such a disorder is sabotaging efforts directed at getting him or her to work or socialize at an expected level. Rather than outright refusing a job assignment, for example, a passive-aggressive carpenter might arrive late, forget his tools, work deliberately slowly or sloppily or become sulky and irritable.

Usually, such people think they are doing better work than they really are and get very angry when others make useful suggestions about how their performance might be improved. They tend to be critical of those in authority.

Dependent Personality Disorder

The essential feature of *dependent personality disorder* is overreliance on others. People with this disorder seem to need an excessive amount of advice and reassurance and often defer important decisions in their lives to those around them. They tend to doubt their own opinions and judgments and, therefore, find it difficult to initiate projects independently.

One of my patients had felt "lost" until she met and married her husband. Thereafter, she considered him to be her "sole source of strength." She could plan her day and socialize in limited ways, but only because she knew that she had the support and company of her husband. He made all the family decisions, and when he was at work and unavailable to advise her, she felt extremely unsure of herself, vulnerable and on edge. His death left her intensely angry and depressed. She eventually formed a small number of superficial friendships, but was petrified that something she said or did would offend these individuals and, therefore, generally kept her thoughts to herself.

My patient's fear of being alone was typical of those people with dependent personality disorder. Such people go to great lengths to avoid being isolated or abandoned, whether physically or emotionally. In order to keep others involved with them, they may do things that require self-sacrifice, even if they find those things unpleasant or frankly distasteful. They might repeatedly volunteer to cut a neighbor's lawn or clean a friend's house. Rather than risk being ostracized, they might pretend to agree with beliefs that they actually do not espouse.

Because they lack confidence in what they think and what they do, criticism or disapproval cuts such people to the core.

Obsessive-Compulsive Personality Disorder

... the patient is troubled by problems at work. He is known as the hardest-driving member of a hard-driving law firm. He was the youngest full partner in the firm's history, and is famous for being able to handle many cases at the same time. Lately, he finds himself increasingly unable to keep up. He is too proud to turn down a new case, and too much of a perfectionist to be satisfied with the quality of work performed by his assistants.... When assignments get backed up, he cannot decide which to address first, starts making schedules for himself and his staff, but then is unable to meet them and works 15 hours a day....

The patient discusses his children as if they were mechanical dolls, but also with a clear underlying affection. He describes his wife as a "suitable mate."... He is punctilious in his manners and dress and slow and ponderous in his speech, dry and humorless, with a stubborn determination to get his point across.

This case illustrates many of the features of *obsessive-compulsive personality disorder*. Unlike patients with *obsessive-compulsive disorder* (see Chapter 12), these patients do not struggle against intrusive thoughts and behavioral rituals. Rather, they are preoccupied with orderliness and perfectionism.

Such people show excessive devotion to work and seem overly conscientious, scrupulous and preoccupied with details and rules. In spite of devoting a great deal of time and energy to a task, they may become mired in the intricacies of it, or unable to share the responsibility for it, and simply never get it done.

In addition, persons with obsessive-compulsive personality disorder tend to be emotionally restricted, as if showing or expressing strong feelings would be too messy for them.

Because they want to hold on to things, they may accumulate old clothing or other belongings long after these items are useful to them. They may be stingy with their time or money.

Are Personality Disorders Inherited?

Psychiatry is still struggling to understand whether personality traits and personality disorders can be transmitted genetically. The evidence for a genetic factor is most convincing in antisocial, paranoid and schizotypal patients. People who have first-degree relatives with schizophrenia, for example, are more likely to develop schizotypal personality features, even if they are adopted and raised by "healthy" families.

Investigators have noted that some of the symptoms of these and other personality disorders seem similar to the symptoms of major mental illnesses. Not only do people with schizotypal personality disorder have characteristics in common with schizophrenic patients, but those with avoidant personality disorder suffer with symptoms that recall anxiety disorders. And those with borderline personality disorder often experience severe mood instability. It may be, then, that many cases of what we now call "personality disorders" actually represent subtle (and, perhaps, equally heritable) disorders of thought, perception, anxiety or mood.

This theory is also supported by the observation that individuals with a personality disorder are vulnerable to developing much more severe symptoms—such as frank psychosis—when under stress.

Personality Disorders and the Brain

Although personality disorders have generally been understood in psychodynamic terms (see the third section of this book), we should not be surprised that researchers have uncovered associated brain abnormalities. We have known for decades, after all, that temporal lobe epilepsy or damage to the brain's frontal lobes can radically alter a person's character (see Chapter 9).

The link between personality disorders and the nervous system has been strengthened and greatly refined by research showing that people with personality disorders often have neurochemical abnormalities similar to those found in patients with major mental illnesses. These include, for example, increased levels of a chemical called *homovanillic acid* (one of the breakdown products of dopamine) in both schizophrenic patients and those diagnosed with schizotypal personality disorder. Patients with borderline personality disorder often have abnormalities of sleep and of the *noradrenergic* (i.e., involving norepinephrine) *neurotransmitter system*, both of which are often amiss in mood disorders, as well. Dysfunction in the *serotonergic system* has been implicated in antisocial personality disorder.

Our evolving understanding of personality disorders illustrates the importance of bringing both medical and psychological resources to bear in alleviating our patients' suffering. When faced with an individual with severe borderline personality disorder, for example, we try to understand the psychological roots of the disorder. We will want to know whether that individual was neglected or abused as a child. We hope, through psychotherapy, to reshape the nonproductive patterns of thought and behavior that have resulted. But we also keep one eye on the brain, knowing that such a patient may have an underlying neurochemical imbalance and, if so, may find certain medicines helpful in coping with the demands of the world around him or her.

Medicines for Personality Disorders

Medications have a growing, but still limited, role in the treatment of personality disorders. When they are used, it is generally for the relief of psychosis, mood lability or symptoms of anxiety. Low-dose antipsychotic medications, for example, are sometimes helpful to patients with severe symptoms of paranoid, schizoid or schizotypal personality disorder. Some borderline patients benefit from antidepressants and mood stabilizers (such as lithium). Antianxiety medicines can be useful in relieving some of the distress accompanying dependent personality disorder.

The treatment of personality disorders with medicines is a relatively new area of research, certain to yield more specific strategies in the future.

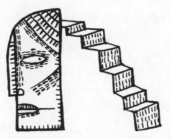

14

Eating Disorders

"An Unconquerable Passion"

The following reflections of a young woman with an eating disorder were shared with her German physician, Moshe Wulff (1878–1971). Wulff included them in a paper he delivered before the German Psychoanalytic Society on April 12, 1932. They have been translated by Albert Stunkard, M.D.

I don't always eat in the same way. Sometimes there occurs to me a particular mental state and then I eat a great deal. I call this condition the "spiritually degenerate condition of a person who has fallen to a low moral level." As soon as I begin to eat very much I am possessed by a bad mood, deep despair and hopelessness, apathetic indifference, complete loss of will, no desires, no joy. I don't work, become completely apathetic and very sleepy. I eat a great deal, almost all day long. And then I become very fat, as if swollen, as if edematous. My appearance changes, I look completely different. I don't want to get dressed and wear only old dirty clothes, preferably only an old bathrobe, don't comb my hair, wash very little and insufficiently. . . . In this condition eating is an unconquerable passion to which I succumb and that I cannot fight against. I have compared myself to an alcoholic, an addict. Sweets and baked goods have a particularly powerful attraction for me. . . .

. . . One evening it is completely unbearable—and the next morning I get up as if transformed, don't know why, and feel that I am fresh, lively, energetic; I feel well. Then I eat very little. In a very good spiritual condition I eat absolutely nothing. . . . However, if I once eat my fill, there follows remorse, anxiety, and despondency; I feel that once again

I have fallen to a low moral level, believe that I have spoiled everything, promise myself that I will never do it again. I make a powerful effort of will to come out of this condition, and I am in complete despair if I am not successful! And I remain in this condition as long as I am not able to abstain from food, thereby freeing myself from these tormenting feelings and bringing back the good elevated condition of abstinence. . . .

Bulimia and Anorexia

Wulff's patient suffered with *bulimia nervosa*, a condition marked by a persistent overconcern with body shape and weight, recurrent episodes of binge eating, a feeling of helplessness to control food intake, and vigorous attempts to prevent weight gain (whether by vomiting, vigorous exercise, use of laxatives or diuretics, strict dieting or fasting).[†]

Bulimia generally begins in adolescence or young adulthood. It strikes females approximately ten times more often than males.

People with bulimia feel driven to *binge* on junk foods rich in carbohydrates. Having done so, they feel guilty and embarrassed and attempt to rid themselves of the calories by, for example, making themselves vomit (called *purging*). They often attempt to hide their behavior from others, including friends, family and physicians. Because a bulimic individual's weight may not vary dramatically, his or her condition can easily go undetected.

Patients with bulimia often suffer with low mood and tend to show impulsive behaviors, including shoplifting, alcohol or drug use, and suicide attempts. Interest in sexual relationships is usually decreased.

Bulimia may become a chronic condition, can wax and wane, or can disappear completely after a period of several months.

Anorexia nervosa remains the most well-known eating disorder. In this condition, patients refuse to maintain normal body weight. They have an intense fear of becoming fat and, even though they are obviously thin, "see" themselves as overweight. In females, the disorder leads to *amenorrhea*, the absence of menstrual cycles.

[†]The complete DSM-III-R diagnostic criteria for bulimia nervosa and anorexia nervosa can be found in Appendixes F and G, respectively.

Anorexia usually begins in teenage girls who are slightly overweight (or feel that they are). Like bulimia, it is approximately ten times more common in females than males. After starting to diet, patients become preoccupied with weight loss and may resort to extreme methods, such as fasting while on vigorous exercise regimens, to achieve quick results.

Anorexic individuals may be at increased risk for mood disorders and sometimes suffer from obsessive-compulsive symptoms, as well. Many of them develop bulimia and begin to binge and purge.

Symptoms may end abruptly, continue to fluctuate for many years or proceed inexorably to starvation and death. Studies have shown that between 5 and 12 percent of patients die from the condition.

Are Eating Disorders Inherited?

It is unclear to what extent, if any, bulimia and anorexia nervosa can be inherited. Some studies have shown that if one identical twin has bulimia or anorexia, the other twin is also at high risk for developing the condition. The likelihood of two *nonidentical* twins both having an eating disorder was shown to be lower, indicating that genetic "closeness" was a determining factor.

In addition, researchers have found that patients with bulimia or anorexia are also likely to suffer with mood disorders or to have family histories that include close relatives with depression. This has led to the theory that eating disorders and mood disorders might be coexisting or related conditions, perhaps inherited together.

Other scientific investigators, however, have disputed these findings. Their studies have shown no genetic risk factor for either bulimia or anorexia and no link between these conditions and mood disorders.

Eating Disorders, Medicines and the Brain

Studies of patients with bulimia and anorexia have revealed a variety of hormonal and neurochemical abnormalities. Some of these are caused by malnutrition itself. Others, however, remain unexplained. Both the serotonergic and noradrenergic neurotransmitter systems may be involved.

Individual, group and behavioral psychotherapies are the mainstays of treatment (see third section of this book) for eating disorders. In addition, some bulimic patients benefit from treatment with either a tricyclic antidepressant, a monoamine oxidase inhibitor or a serotonin reuptake inhibitor, all of which are described in Chapter 11.

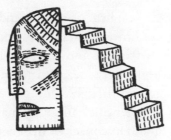

A Note on the Brain and the Mind

15

> It was, of course, a grand and impressive thing to do, to mistrust the obvious, and to pin one's faith in things which could not be seen!
>
> —Galen (A.D. 129–199) *On the Natural Faculties*

Psychiatry is a medical specialty with deep spiritual and philosophical roots. One can even imagine that had Freud developed his interests in emotions after studying theology, rather than neurology, psychoanalysis might have evolved into a quasi-religious order based on the individual's deeply rooted connection to fellow humans; the power of empathy to heal both illness and depravity; and the meanings of dreams, voices and visions. This "church of psychiatry," with practitioners interested in the mind but not the brain, would, tragically, have missed the biological keys to relieving many forms of human suffering.

Freud was, of course, a physician. His theories and their offshoots have found a home in medical offices, clinics and hospitals. Like churches, these environments are not without beliefs, rituals and preconceptions. Medical training, for example, emphasizes the importance of statistical proofs and physical evidence. To a certain extent, it cultivates a distrust of "gut feelings." It is testimony to the power of Freud's thematic, intuitive findings that their roots have continued to hold in this kind of soil.

The tension between the medical profession and ideas such as the ego and the Oedipus complex, however, has increased as medical technology has evolved. With machines and research methods available to visualize and characterize brain tissue, with more and more medicines on hand to combat disordered thoughts and perceptions, a new skepticism has focused on less "scientific" interpersonal techniques that are based in empathy, insight and unconscious dynamics.

The cases of Oliver, Maria and Samuel (described in the first section of this book), however, show that biological and psychological approaches can be complementary ways of understanding and treating the same disorders. The healing power of helping someone understand his or her life may be palpable and genuine, yet utterly untranslatable into the language of genetics, neurotransmitters or synapses.

Author Robert Pirsig, writing about biology's influence on anthropology, has used an intriguing analogy to a word processor and novel. It is also a useful way to think of the brain's relationship to the life story— and to the mind:

> Certainly the novel cannot exist in the computer without a parallel pattern of voltages to support it. But that does not mean that the novel is an expression or property of those voltages. . . . It can reside in a notebook but it is not composed of or possessed by the ink and paper. It can reside in the brain of a programmer, but even here it is neither composed of this brain nor possessed by it. . . .
>
> Trying to explain social moral patterns in terms of inorganic chemistry patterns is like trying to explain the plot of a word-processor novel in terms of the computer's electronics. You can't do it. You can see how the circuits make the novel possible, but they do not provide a plot for the novel.

Thinking About
the Mind

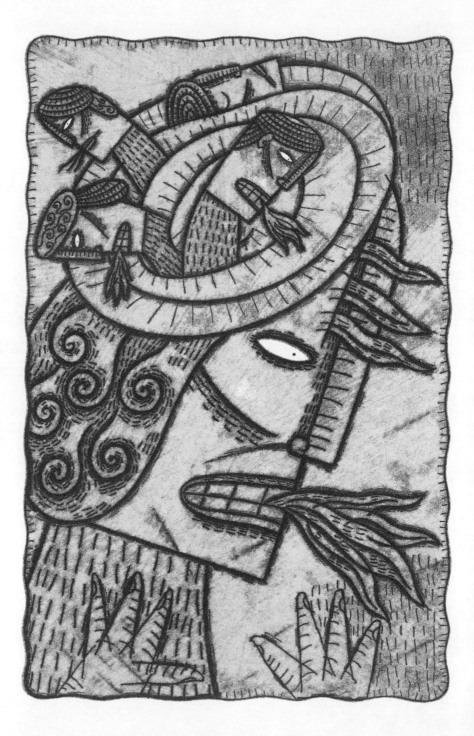

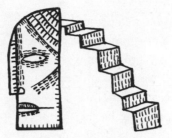

16

The Maggot

Toni had seemed angry from the moment I introduced myself to her and her mother in the waiting room. She was thirty years old—a single mother with a ten-year-old daughter of her own—but now, having plopped down into the chair opposite mine, sighing annoyedly and staring at the floor, she seemed more like an irate child. The fact that her mother had accompanied her to her appointment added to her childlike presence. After a full minute of silence she glanced at me, chuckled to herself, shook her head and focused on the ceiling.

I worried that an emotionally distant psychotherapeutic stance would alienate her. "We certainly seem to be hitting it off," I joked.

She fought against the slightest hint of a smile, then turned to me with a scowl. "As soon as I saw you come into the clinic," she said, "I told my mother, 'I certainly hope that one's not my doctor. He's a maggot.'"

Since Toni and I had never met before, I read her strong emotional reaction to me as *transference*, the irrational displacement onto the therapist of the patient's feelings about other important figures in his or her life. Part of my job is to serve as a lightning rod for these displaced emotions. If I can inspire trust, patients may be able to play out their unconscious conflicts with me, slowly understanding and making peace with them.

Portions of this chapter were first published in *The Washington Post*.

"What do you mean by 'a maggot'?" I asked.

"You know. A liar, a cheat, a snake. A maggot's a lowlife."

"And how can you recognize a maggot so quickly?"

"I know one when I see one," she said curtly. She seemed to relax a bit. "I attract them. *They* find *me*."

Maggots, of course, are the larvae of insects and are usually found in decaying matter. Toni's feeling that maggots were attracted to her made me wonder whether she not only felt victimized, but as if she was dirty or wasting away. Her other symptoms fit with this theme. She was suffering from a severe depression (which had left her nearly housebound) and bulimia. Unable to sleep past the early morning hours, having lost twenty pounds, she appeared tired, pale and gaunt.

"What other maggots have you met up with?" I asked during our second meeting.

"Dozens," she quickly answered. "You could put me in a room with a hundred guys, and if there was one lowlife there, I'd somehow manage to shack up with him."

Each of Toni's relationships had begun with an initial period of powerful infatuation. She would miss early and obvious signs that she was being drawn to someone of questionable character. If friends told her, for example, that her new love interest was a philanderer, drug abuser or criminal, she would dismiss the evidence as lies, rumors or "ancient history." If his last girlfriend confided that she had been brutalized, Toni would reject the warning as "pure jealousy." Almost without exception, romance turned to sex within two dates. And each time a lover turned out to be emotionally or physically abusive to her she felt shocked, violated and defective.

A pattern of engaging in abusive relationships like the ones Toni described brings out the sleuth in a psychiatrist. What, I wondered, was the driving force from her past that would lead her to be attracted to, then revulsed by, man after man? What connected that compulsive dynamic with her disordered eating and her depression? Why should her symptoms be worse now, rather than a year ago or two years hence? What chapter in her earlier life story was so powerfully influencing the evolving plot?

"I'm sure you'll do it to me, too," she said.

"Do what?" I asked.

"Set me up."

"How so?"

She shrugged. "I don't know. Maybe I'll come in here one day for an appointment, and they'll tell me you don't work here anymore. You took off. Who knows what could happen?"

Toni's fear that I would abandon her (together with the fact that she continued to live with her parents and that her mother was again waiting outside my office) made me wonder what other difficulties she had had with separation. She told me that as a young girl she had played sick or refused to attend school for several days at a time. She recalled worrying about her mother's safety on those occasions when her father, an "abusive" alcoholic, had been drinking.

Would I disappoint her? I anticipated that during Toni's therapy she would unconsciously be moved to test my reliability, again and again. *"Who knows what could happen?"* she had said.

Other troubling thoughts had come to my mind. First, Toni's description of her father as abusive, together with her depression, eating disorder, low self-esteem and separation anxiety, made me wonder whether he had abused her emotionally, physically or sexually.

In psychodynamic theory, depression and self-abusive behavior can be caused when a patient turns feelings of anger and aggression inward. Redirecting rage meant for another person protects the real target (a father, for example, toward whom a child feels murderous rage) at the expense of the self. Was her father the first maggot in her life?

I had also become aware of my own physical attraction to Toni. This was essential data because my role as her psychiatrist clearly put me in a position of both trust and authority. Almost like a father. I wondered whether our therapeutic interaction was beginning to mirror earlier abuse she had suffered.

What about me, I asked myself, could put me at risk for promoting such a dynamic, rather than interpreting and helping her to understand it? Anticipating these pitfalls is the best strategy for avoiding them. I must remain aware that I come to the clinic with my own life history, my own buried conflicts. There is the danger that I will play those issues out in the context of the therapy—unconsciously writing a script for the patient. I resolved to be alert for any *countertransference*, my projection onto Toni of emotions transplanted from other relationships in my life.

On the surface of things our therapy consisted of two people who had met for two hours. But our relationship really embodied unconscious traces of both our pasts—emotions left over from hours, a year or a decade before our first meetings.

None of my attention to the workings of the mind had distracted me from thinking about the brain. I knew that Toni's family included other members who had suffered with addictions, mood disorders and eating disorders. I was aware of the possible genetic link between her depression and her bulimia. I had tested her thyroid function and found it to be normal. I had begun the medication I thought would be best for her. But the fact that I believed that Toni's neurotransmitters might well be amiss and that a medication might relieve some of her symptoms didn't make the dynamics behind those symptoms any less real or important to me. I reminded myself (as I always do) that *every person is sick in his or her own way*.

> . . . You can see how the circuits make the novel possible, but they do
> not provide a plot for the novel.

Toni came to our third meeting alone, without her mother. The full weight of Toni's depression seemed to be bearing down upon her. She had not left the house at all during the week following our previous meeting. She had binged and purged relentlessly. Rather than seeming irritable, she looked terribly sad. After a few minutes of silence she began to cry.

"Do you have an idea where those tears are coming from?" I asked.

She shook her head. "I can't feel anything, anymore. It's my daughter's eleventh birthday, and I can't even be happy about that. I didn't make her a party. Nothing. I should never have been a mother."

The connection between Toni's tears, her daughter's birthday and her doubt about how good a mother she could be made me wonder whether age eleven had been a traumatic time for her—a time, perhaps, when her own mother had failed her.

"Why do you mention your daughter's birthday?" I asked.

"I don't know," she said. "I don't think that has anything to do with anything." She was sobbing heavily now. "There is something I haven't told you, though."

"Only one thing?" I smiled.

She took a deep breath and wiped away her tears. "I haven't told anyone."

I nodded.

"My father used to visit my room after my mother went to bed," she whispered. "He used to touch me."

"When did this happen?" I asked.

"It started when I was eleven," she said. She looked confused, then genuinely surprised at the coincidence. "Eleven," she whispered, shaking her head and again beginning to cry.

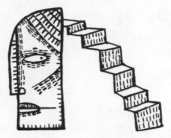

17

The Workings
of the Human Mind

To know that what is impenetrable to us really exists, manifesting itself as the highest wisdom and the most radiant beauty, which our dull facilities can comprehend only in the most primitive forms—this knowledge, this feeling, is at the center of true religiousness. In this sense, and in this sense only, I belong to the ranks of the devoutly religious men.

—Albert Einstein *What I Believe* (1930)

After all, psychodynamics is no more than a system of metaphors, a metapsychology devised to explain the unknown, and it is not readily susceptible to experimental proof.

—George Vaillant

The evidence that powerful forces beyond the synapse operate in human thought, emotion and relationships has been at hand for hundreds of years. During the eighteenth century, Franz Anton Mesmer (1734–1815) effectively treated thousands of patients with what he called the magnetic pass. He would sit opposite a patient, their knees touching, and sweep his hands repeatedly from the patient's head to midsection. The patient would experience a warm wave washing over his or her body and would lapse into a convulsion. Upon awakening, the patient's symptoms—whether paralysis or blindness or terrible anxiety—

were often gone. Mesmer's theory was that his treatment had restored
the free flow of a magnetized internal fluid through his patients' organs.

Mesmer's treatment was discredited when it was shown that patients
improved equally if they simply *believed* they had been magnetized, even
if no procedure had been performed. But why, then, did Mesmer's patients recover at all? What, indeed, had been the matter with them?

Over the next century, other scientists, including the English surgeon
James Braid (1795–1860) and the French neurologist Jean Charcot
(1825–1893), found that the clinician's *suggestion* that a patient ought
to recover was often enough to cure that person. And under the structured form of suggestion called *hypnosis*, they observed that many patients
with unusual symptoms spoke of long-forgotten traumatic experiences that
seemed thematically connected to their suffering. One such patient, of the
French physician Pierre Janet (1859–1947), was a woman who was afraid
of the color red. She insisted that she had no idea why this should be.
Under hypnosis, however, she vividly described her father's funeral, particularly a bunch of red flowers that had been laid on his casket.

The theory of *dissociation* grew from such observations. The theory
held that mental functions could be split off from consciousness, leaving
the individual completely unaware of them. Rather than remaining buried and inert, however, these banished perceptions, thoughts and memories were transformed and resurrected—as symptoms. Someone who
witnessed terrible violence, for instance, might become blind (the disability then being called *hysterical* blindness). A man who had been
injured in a war and who, unconsciously, wanted to remain safely behind the lines of battle might fall victim to hysterical paralysis. When
traumas were sufficient to split off many elements of the persona, what
we now call *multiple personality disorder* could result.

Sigmund Freud (1856–1939) and Josef Breuer (1842–1925) were the
first to assert that helping patients to bring these buried thoughts, memories and emotions into consciousness was the means by which they
could be cured.

Freud postulated that the mind's structure consisted of what he called
id, *ego* and *superego*.

The id is the part of the mind that contains our unconscious and
instinctive desires and *drives*, such as sexual and aggressive impulses.

The ego is the mind's negotiator, helping the individual to adapt the desires and drives of the id to the demands of the external world. To achieve an orderly discharge of the unwieldy energy stored in the id, the ego utilizes perception, control of the body's musculature, language, logical thought and a wide range of *unconscious defense mechanisms* (of which more will be said later).

Finally, the superego develops from the ego and comes to embody the individual's ethics and social standards. It is the location of the conscience and the *ego ideals*—strongly held notions of what kind of people we wish to be. As Freud wrote:

> The long period of childhood, during which the growing human being lives in dependence upon his parents, leaves behind it a precipitate, which forms within his ego a special agency in which this parental influence is prolonged. It has received the name of *superego*. In so far as this superego is differentiated from the ego or opposed to it, it constitutes a third force which the ego must take into account.

The ego, then, is often in a position of mediating between the drives of the id and the moral constraints of the superego. A young woman on a first date, for example, might be powerfully attracted (id) to her young man, worry that acting on her desire would be immoral (superego), and decide (ego) that light fondling will be the limit she imposes on herself and her date pending a more extended courtship. To enact her decision she might utilize other ego functions, such as speech ("We should wait"), sensation (feeling her date's touch under the hem of her dress) and muscular activity (moving her date's hand away).

Ego Defense Mechanisms

Central to understanding a psychoanalytic theory of the mind is the concept of ego mechanisms of defense. These are mental gymnastics that the ego employs (whether in health or illness) in order to protect the individual from stress, allow him or her to function in society, and cultivate some degree of inner peace. Usually, the defenses involve altering one's perception of reality.

Ego defenses are essential to psychological well-being. Without them, the full weight of the stress of our lives and the raw energy of the id might crush us. We often need to temporarily deny certain facts, for example, in order to respond rationally and slowly come to terms with them.

Sometimes, however, the ego's defenses can cause symptoms we regard as *disorders*. For example, Oliver's belief that his daughter had been kidnapped and replaced by a masquerading double (see Chapter 1) could be thought of as a defense (in this case, a psychotic distortion of reality) against the pain of her abandoning him in a time of need.

Maria's burning feet (see Chapter 4) could be understood as the *conversion* of her grief at her grandson's absence into a physical symptom.

And Toni's depression and disordered eating (see Chapter 16) could be conceived of partly as a defense (here, *turning against the self*) against feelings of anger and aggression toward her father that were considered by her ego to be potentially too destructive. The ego might unconsciously "reason" in this way: "You would like to destroy your father [the id's directive] for his behavior when you were eleven years old, but this is an unacceptable act [proscribed by the superego]. Therefore, you will turn that anger inward, depleting your murderous emotions and rendering you fatigued and less capable of such behavior." This kind of unconscious process could also result in suicide, the ultimate pathological redirecting of murderous rage against the self.

While the symptoms resulting from the defense mechanisms in these three cases would constitute *disorders* (perhaps reflecting ego *defects*), they are also close cousins of the dynamic and healthy coping strategies we all use. As George Vaillant has written:

> Whereas nineteenth-century medical phenomenologists viewed pus, fever, pain, and coughing as evidence of disease, twentieth-century pathophysiologists regard these symptoms as evidence of the body's healthy efforts to cope with physical or infectious insult. In parallel fashion much of what modern psychiatric phenomenologists classify as disorders according to the *Diagnostic and Statistical Manual of Mental Disorders*, third edition (DSM-III) can be reclassified by those with a more psychodynamic viewpoint as manifestations of the ego's adaptive efforts to cope with psychological stress.

A Potpourri of Ego Defenses

Repression

According to psychoanalytic theory, repression is the ego's ability to banish unacceptable thoughts, emotions, fantasies or memories into the unconscious and keep them there. It is the universal mechanism, for example, responsible for our "forgetting" most of our early years. It is also the means by which we exclude sexual feelings for family members from consciousness.

Repression can lead to cloudy memories of, or complete amnesia for, traumatic events in an individual's life. In Toni's case, it could explain her "forgetting" why her daughter's eleventh birthday might be a stressful time for her.

Isolation

The ego uses isolation to unconsciously split an idea or event away from the painful or frightening emotions associated with it. The process allows reporters to objectively and painstakingly chronicle terrible tragedies and allows doctors to work amid suffering without being paralyzed by grief.

A victim of a violent crime may arrive in the emergency room, for example, showing little emotion and talking calmly about the need for more police officers and the possible deterrent value of the death penalty. The trauma has been unconsciously cleansed of its personal impact and turned into a relatively sterile discussion of issues.

When isolation is excessive, it can become a way of life, leaving people habitually out of touch with their emotions. It can also lead to obsessive characteristics, such as preoccupation with details, rules and work, to the exclusion of any attention to feelings.

Denial

Denial is the disavowal of facts that, if acknowledged, would cause emotional pain, anxiety or conflict. It is the unconscious force that leads individuals, for example, to reflexively reject news of a loved one's death as untrue or to ignore serious warning signs of illness. Usually, denial is transient, and the person, in more or less timely fashion, comes to see things for what they really are.

In some cases, however, denial is more tenacious. In its extreme form, it can even lead to delusional thinking. A woman whose child is still-born, for example, may utterly reject that fact and become unshakably attached to the idea that the baby has been abducted.

Displacement

In displacement, troubling emotions, ideas or desires associated with one person or situation are transferred to a substitute. A man who is unconsciously attracted to his teenage daughter, for example, may be moved to have an affair with a much younger woman or to visit a young prostitute. A woman struggling for independence from her mother might unconsciously displace her frustrations into an argument with a female supervisor at work. Toni had displaced her anger at abusive men, including her father—"maggots"—onto me.

Displacement is thought to play a critical role in the development of anxiety disorders. If a young boy, for example, is driving over a bridge with his father when his father suffers a heart attack, the emotions associated with that event may, years later, turn up as a displaced fear of heights.

Turning Against the Self

Turning against the self is the inward displacement of emotions felt toward someone else. When the expression of explosive rage or aggression is seen by the ego as unacceptable, it can essentially implode those feelings, sometimes causing severe psychiatric symptoms. We have already spoken, for example, of Toni's depression as the possible result of "anger turned inwards."

This defense mechanism, when operating at pathologic proportions, may explain why a disproportionate number of victims of childhood abuse go on to suicide.

Negation

When certain feelings are too stressful to express directly, they may be vented through an ego defense called negation. This involves speaking of one's *true* feelings as another's hypothesis, and then rejecting it. For example, someone who is devastated by a spouse's infidelity might complain, "If you think this is tearing me up inside, if you think I'm all worried about whether I'm still attractive to you, then you're more arrogant than I thought. Actually, all I feel toward you right now is pity."

Reaction Formation

> The lady doth protest too much, methinks.
>
> —Shakespeare *Hamlet*

Reaction formation can color a person's entire life history. It is a process by which a person's true but uncomfortable feelings, attitudes and wishes are unconsciously replaced by their opposites. For example, a man with doubts about his masculinity may unconsciously exorcise any bit of femininity from his appearance, speech and behavior. He might develop a reputation for stoicism or even become a boxer.

Ernest Hemingway, for example, is said to have been dressed by his mother in female clothing when he was a boy. This kind of confusing, stressful experience could have unconsciously contributed to his developing into a "man's man."

Someone who actually yearns to be dependent on others may live by himself or herself, reject help from family and friends and come to be seen (misunderstood, actually) by the community as a loner.

Toni made a great deal of her respect for her mother, whom she said had never let her down. During therapy, however, it became apparent that Toni suspected that her mother had known of the abuse she was suffering. Toni was terrified of expressing the anger and betrayal she felt. "If I were to lose her," she said, "I'd have no one left."

Projection

Projection is an ego defense mechanism in which feelings unacceptable to the self are unconsciously rejected and attributed to others. If a person suspects himself or herself of being weak, corrupt or evil, for example, he or she may attribute that quality to another person or group of people. This is how scapegoats are created. Hitler, it might be theorized, had deeply rooted problems with low self-esteem which he projected onto an entire race of people he called "inferior."

To use a more common example, a person who is unconsciously shielding himself or herself from feelings of depression may comment that a friend "seems depressed" or "looks sad."

Anxiety-provoking impulses can also lead to projection. A man who has unconscious violent tendencies may feel that others mean to harm *him*. Psychoanalytic theory predicts that such a person might even become paranoid or hear imaginary voices of passersby threatening him.

Identification

Identification is the unconscious incorporation into oneself of qualities, beliefs or behaviors that belong to significant people in one's life. It is responsible for friends beginning to speak alike and for students unconsciously adopting the patterns of dress of favorite teachers. An example from my personal experience is that, midway through my psychiatry residency, I purchased an expensive leather briefcase at a local shop. It cost more than I really wanted to spend. Not until three weeks later did I notice that my supervisor, a role model of mine, had been carrying the exact same briefcase since I had known him.

Identification also operates to take the edge off the grief of a loved one's loss by internalizing something about that person. A deceased politician's wife who runs for his political office may be doing so, in part, to preserve her comforting internal image of him.

It has also been recognized that fear can be unconsciously channeled into *identification with the aggressor*, a phenomenon theorized to be responsible for hostages coming to "believe" in the cause of their captors. By psychologically adopting the alien beliefs and values of aggressors, the anxiety of being at their mercy is blunted.

Regression

When a person is faced with an anxiety-provoking situation, he or she may retreat to patterns of thought and behavior characteristic of an earlier developmental stage. A woman emotionally unprepared for the stress and responsibilities of child rearing, for example, might become depressed after giving birth and move back into her parents' home to be cared for.

Regression may be responsible for a wide range of psychiatric disorders, especially those that result in frequent hospital stays (during which many of the patient's needs are provided for by staff).

One patient I treated had been a successful businessman who, faced with stresses related to his sexuality, became afraid to leave the house. He "preferred" instead to stay in his bedroom, cuddling with a stuffed bear. His mother would drive from a neighboring town to bring him his dinner each evening.

Conversion

In conversion, psychological stresses or conflicts that would otherwise give rise to feelings of anxiety are instead channeled (i.e., converted) into physical symptoms or disabilities. It is the force that is thought to be responsible when children, having been teased by their classmates or threatened by the class bully, feel too sick the next day to attend school.

The role of conversion in producing bodily symptoms may explain why Mesmer's magnetic pass, perhaps by virtue of his own supportive manner, was able to rid patients of so many "physical" ailments (ailments like Maria's burning feet). It is also possible that this ego defense is sometimes neutralized by the emotional excitement stimulated by faith healing.

Losing Balance

According to a psychoanalytic model, mental health relies on the maintenance of an emotional dynamic equilibrium. The ego, confronted with the drives of the id, the stresses of the external world and the social guidelines of the superego, strikes an infinite number of psychological bargains to lower anxiety and keep the person "balanced." Many of these bargains are struck through the arbitration of the ego's mechanisms of defense. In the healthy mind, these defenses alter reality and sculpt the individual's personality just enough to let him or her cope and adjust gently to an ever-changing environment.

Trouble starts when the ego, whether due to its inherent weaknesses (sometimes stemming from problems in early childhood development) or overwhelming environmental stresses, either resorts to "unhealthy" defenses (such as psychosis) or fails to contain the unwieldy instinctive drives of the id.

In a man, for example, whose early life experience (perhaps marked by an alcoholic and unreliable mother) led to anxiety about being cared for adequately, the ego defense mechanism of reaction formation may intervene. Such a man might grow up to be overly independent, a rugged individualist who makes a great deal of needing no one's help to get along.

In a woman whose father is sexually intrusive—attempting, for example, to watch her undress repeatedly during early adolescence—the ego defense of isolation might lead her to be chaste and a compulsive worker, to the exclusion of anxiety-provoking sexual feelings and romantic relationships.

If life events, however, increase the demands on the ego, havoc can ensue. The self-sufficient man, for example, faced with new professional tasks that demand teamwork, may be unable to ask for help. He is trapped within his character structure and, because of strain on the ego, may become depressed, experiencing a fall in self-esteem, impaired sleep and decreased concentration. By the ego resorting to the defense of projection, he might accuse others of being unreasonably dependent on him, because he is so fearful of being dependent on them. And rather than confront his own painful longing for support, his ego might even defend itself through a psychotic distortion of reality, leaving him paranoid that others are sabotaging his projects.

The obsessive, workaholic woman, desiring a family, may marry. Faced with the strain of her husband's expectations of having marital relations, she may become anxious and fearful. Rather than confronting her troubling and conflicted feelings about sex (and her father), her ego may employ the additional defense of conversion, making her experience terrible vaginal pain that precludes sexual intercourse.

Vulnerabilities

No themes are so human as those that reflect for us, out of the confusion of life, the close connection of bliss and bale, of the things that help with the things that hurt, so dangling before us forever that bright hard medal, of so strange an alloy, one face of which is somebody's right and ease and the other somebody's pain and wrong.

—Henry James Preface to "What Maisie Knew"

What should be clear is that people experience events differently. Not only do we each develop individual psychological strategies to negotiate the twists and turns of life, but we will differ on whether an event—be it a job change, marriage or an illness in the family—represents a relatively minor detour in the road, a treacherous curve or a complete impasse.

The roots of the Achilles' heels leading to psychiatric disorders are sometimes found in our earliest years when we are, according to psychoanalytic thinking, passing through critical phases of psychosexual development, learning about our internal and external environments. These phases include periods when we are exploring and deriving sustenance, relief or pleasure from our oral, anal and genital functions.

Not all psychiatrists believe that this particular blueprint for development really explains adult character traits. It is presented here as one example of life story reasoning.

Oral Phase

The oral phase of development runs from birth to approximately eighteen months of age. It is during this time that the infant is focused on the mouth as a region associated with the relief of hunger, with pleasure (sucking, swallowing) and with the expression of aggressive drives (spitting, biting).

Healthy development during this phase is theorized to be related to the ability to trust others and to engage with others in mutually supportive relationships. Trauma during this phase, on the other hand, can lead to demanding or dependent personality traits. Such individuals may also be overly optimistic, pessimistic or envious.

Some patients with borderline personality disorder, for example, are thought, according to this model, to have been inadequately nurtured during this critical period, leaving them without the emotional resources to have balanced relationships with others. They often lack the ability to trust, suspect that others mean to cause them pain, and interpret normal interpersonal distance as standoffishness or abandonment.

Anal Phase

The anal phase of psychosexual development lasts from ages eighteen months to approximately three years. During this time, the child is achieving better control over his or her bodily function of voiding feces, a glimmer of personal independence and autonomy. This process, however, includes toilet training by parents. Struggles over control of voiding—when and where it will take place—naturally arise. The child learns that he or she elicits praise or scorn from mother and father, makes them proud or distressed, depending on how closely his or her voiding behavior matches their expectations.

When these normal struggles between child and parents are met with excessive parental anger, disappointment or an overly strict and ritualized program of toilet training, the child may retreat from this experiment in self-control, returning to behavior patterns more typical of the oral phase, such as thumb sucking.

Positive growth during the anal phase is thought to set the stage for independence and autonomy in adulthood. On the other hand, unresolved conflicts during this time may lead to personality traits like ambivalence, excessive concern with orderliness, stubbornness, defiance and sadomasochistic tendencies.

Genital Phase

The genital phase lasts from ages three through five. During this time, the child comes to recognize that there are two different sexes, and his or her genitals (and those of the opposite sex) become the primary focus of interest.

The genital phase includes manifestations of what has come to be known as the *Oedipus complex*—a child's sexual attraction to the parent of opposite sex, along with feelings of envy and aggression toward the parent of the same sex. Boys fantasize, for example, about banishing or doing away with their fathers. Girls fantasize about replacing their mothers and bearing their fathers' children.

Resolving such conflicted feelings necessarily involves repeated frustration of the child's competitive instincts. Gradually (in a healthy family) the child gives up his or her incestuous and hostile wishes (at the behest of the superego) and comes to ally and identify with the parent of the same sex.

According to Freud's theory, excessive turmoil during the genital phase, when such violent and passionate fantasies are alive in the child's mind, can be the foundation of much psychological suffering later in life.

A fifty-year-old patient of mine named Stewart, for example, suffered terrible symptoms of fear and anxiety whenever he felt himself becoming romantically attached to a woman. He could not fight off the sense of impending disaster that repeatedly visited him, complete with heart palpitations, dizziness and sweats. On one occasion, having prepared to propose marriage to a woman at an elegant restaurant, his heart began to beat wildly in his chest, perspiration soaked his shirt, the walls seemed to be closing in on him, and he fled the table. Years later, he had decided to live with another woman, but became intensely (and unjustifiably) suspicious that she was being unfaithful to him and canceled the move. All told, four women with whom he might otherwise have enjoyed lasting relationships ultimately left him because his symptoms interfered so significantly with their lives together.

After several psychotherapy sessions with me, Stewart recalled a traumatic game his mother had repeatedly engaged him in when he was four years old. "She'd say, 'Come here, sweetheart' and hold out her arms," he explained tearfully. "Then, when I did, she'd slap my face good and hard."

It is easy to imagine how, according to psychoanalytic theory, this sadistic childhood "game" could contaminate Stewart's adult relationships. At a point in his life when he was romancing his mother, experiencing all the feelings of desire, guilt and hostility typical of the genital phase of development, he was not permitted to smoothly integrate these conflicts in his mind. His early sexual feelings became unconsciously linked with impending emotional and physical pain. Later in life, real intimacy with a woman unconsciously recalled his mother's bait (open arms) and switch (open hand) abuse and was translated by his ego into anxiety or paranoia, repeatedly forcing him to run away.

The same traumatic experience could as easily have fueled masochistic sexual behavior, in which pleasure can only be achieved if accompanied by physical pain or some form of humiliation.

Another patient of mine, a twenty-two-year-old man named Peter, had become dependent on alcohol. Peter traced the roots of his addiction to his attempts to soothe feelings of anxiety that he had experienced since he was a teenager. The anxiety would come whenever any aggressive feelings visited him. The irritation he felt pushing his way onto a crowded bus, for example, left him terrified of what he might do if his irritation turned to frank anger. His frustration with drivers who cut him off in traffic frightened him to his core. "I'm a loaded gun," he complained. "I could go off and beat the hell out of someone. Worse, *I could kill somebody*. I'm out of control."

Peter's family history included the fact that his father had died when Peter was four years old, well into the oedipal period. This was a time, according to psychoanalytic theory, when Peter would have been struggling with feelings of aggression toward his father and feelings of romantic love for his mother. His young mind may have unconsciously concluded that his wish to rid the family of his father had actually *caused* his father's death, and that his aggressive impulses were unwieldy, potent and extremely dangerous. With the connection between hostility and death (or murder) etched so deeply in his mind, it is no wonder that he remained petrified of losing control of his emotions as an adult.

Keeping Psychiatry's Mind Open

Psycho-analysis is not, like philosophies, a system seeking to grasp the whole universe . . . And, once it is completed, having no room for fresh discoveries or better understanding. On the contrary . . . it gropes its way forward by the help of experience, is always incomplete, and always ready to correct and modify its theories.

—Sigmund Freud

Conceiving of the mind as divided into ego, id and superego and searching out the roots of psychiatric symptoms in oral, anal and genital phases of psychosexual development are powerful ways of understanding a patient's suffering. Using them as conceptual frameworks, psychiatrists can help patients to see how early chapters in their life stories are continuing to influence the evolving plots. In so doing, and for reasons we still cannot translate into neurochemical equations (and may never be able to), their symptoms are often relieved.

Thinkers in psychiatry—Erik Erikson, Heinz Hartmann, Melanie Klein, Heinz Kohut, Abraham Maslow, Jean Piaget, Carl Rogers and many others—have continued to introduce theories about the mind and the self that expand upon, challenge or even completely dismiss Freud's views (which themselves branch far beyond what can be presented in this book). Each theory has in common the goal of helping the patient to find his or her core, best and healthiest self amid storms of past traumas, present stresses, relationships, expectations, goals, losses and the whole host of life events that attend personhood.

The ideas that have been presented are not meant as a rigid, complete or final way to think about the mind. They simply illustrate one kind of reasoning that, coupled with empathy, can heal. No one can say precisely why harnessing words, thoughts, emotions and themes helps to carry patients out of despair, anxiety or even psychosis. To me, however, this should be cause not for worry but for reflection and wonder.

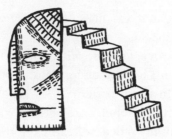

18

Encountering the Mind

The human understanding is like a false mirror, which, receiving rays irregularly, distorts and discolors the nature of things by mingling its own nature with it.

—Francis Bacon (1561–1626) *Novum Organum*

Psychotherapy is a kind of greenhouse in which the ego defenses of both psychiatrist and patient can grow and flower. Part of my job is to bear witness to these unconscious workings of the ego, to strip them of their camouflage, so that patients will have the opportunity to reflect on the emotional conflicts that underlie them.

Central to this therapeutic process is my attention to *transference*, a particular kind of *displacement* (see Chapter 17), wherein the patient unconsciously develops irrational feelings toward the therapist that actually stem from other relationships, often early in life.

Transference is so powerful a force that beginning treatment with a psychiatric patient can make me feel like I am walking onstage in a play, never having read the script and not knowing in what role I have been cast. No wonder that my inclination is to keep quiet and listen.

As already noted, Toni's transference toward me as a "maggot"—another man likely to abuse and abandon her—had begun the moment she first saw me in the clinic (see Chapter 16). Maria, the woman with the burning feet, began to respond to me as if I were her grandson. Oliver, who believed his daughter was missing, wondered whether I was an apparition likely to disappear.

Standing in for abusive fathers, withholding mothers, demanding sons—being a lightening rod for unconscious conflicts—is part of my job. If I can inspire trust, my patients may be able to play out their unresolved emotions through their interactions with me. By examining the dramas unfolding in my office, we can explore these feelings, slowly coming to understand and make peace with them.

Weeks into my work with Toni, for example, I was called to the emergency room and had to cancel one of our meetings. She reacted with great anger.

"You blew me off!" she said later. She tried to retreat from the anger immediately. "You'd really be in trouble if I knew where you lived," she laughed.

"Are you really angry enough to hurt me?" I asked.

"Don't be such a psychiatrist," she taunted. "You're hardly the first guy to stand me up."

"Who was the first?"

She considered the question briefly. "I guess my father."

"And how did he stand you up?"

"He took off for almost a year after I told my mother about his touching me. Disappeared, just like that. I've never thought before how angry that made me."

Examining Toni's anger at me, which I sensed was partly fueled by transference, had allowed her to get in touch with buried feelings about her father—feelings that, left to simmer underground so many years, might have contributed to her depression.

The irrational connections flow both ways. When I feel them toward patients, they are called *countertransference*. I come to the clinic with my own life history, my own buried conflicts. There is the danger that I will play those issues out in the context of therapy—unconsciously writing a script that the patient must act out.

When an older female outpatient of mine considered terminating therapy, for example, it occurred to me that she might be reacting to her son's moving away from home by severing our relationship. Before exploring that possible transference, however, I needed to look at my own feelings. Was my desire to keep the patient in therapy rooted in my intense childhood fear of separation from my mother?

The pushes and pulls of transference and countertransference are much of the reason that some forms of psychotherapy rely on maintaining a rigid structure to the therapeutic relationship. Visits are generally fifty minutes long. They take place in the office. They occur on a regular schedule. Their cost is fixed. The personal life of the therapist may be kept wholly out of the discussion. The doctor's home phone number may be withheld. Any variable introduced into the relationship without consideration may be a contaminant, reflecting the unconscious wishes, needs and fears of either patient or doctor.

A patient who consistently talks past the end of the session, for example, may have a need to exert control. A therapist who gives no real notice of an upcoming vacation may be expressing anger or ambivalence about his or her role as a caregiver.

Even knowing all this, part of me has fantasized about crossing the boundaries of therapy to become the trustworthy father, reliable friend or steadfast lover that my patients need or want. I have wondered whether doing so would alleviate their pain. But that would mean abandoning the role I promised to play at the outset—that of an impartial and empathic observer. It would obliterate a valuable opportunity to demonstrate how the integrity of a relationship can be preserved.

To have real power to heal, psychotherapy must remain a lens to bring life into focus, not a substitute for living.

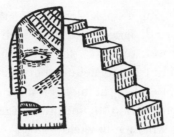

19

Connections

We are most likely to get angry and excited in our opposition to some idea when we ourselves are not quite certain of our own position, and are inwardly tempted to take the other side.

—Thomas Mann *Buddenbrooks* (1901)

Psychiatry would be a simpler profession if all our capacity to heal came from our knowledge of either the brain or the mind. We could listen in just one way to our patients, tuning our ears either to detect the objective symptoms of surging dopamine in the basal ganglia or to hear and feel the pain of unresolved emotional conflicts straining the ego. Our research efforts could hinge entirely on the evolution of technology or on the evolution of interpersonal understanding.

Indeed, the wish for a clearer, more direct road might underlie the infighting between those psychiatrists who insist all mental illness should be understood in terms of abnormal brain chemistry, and others who argue that brain chemistry is nothing but a detour from the real truths about human suffering.

The complexity in psychiatry (and, in my opinion, the ultimate beauty) is a result of the field's diversity of clinical perspectives. We have taken our gifts of knowledge as they have come. We have found power in antidepressants *and* in empathy, in the careful diagnosis of disorders (using DSM-III-R) *and* the painstaking interpretation of individual life stories.

157

This means that treating a single depressed patient can mean listening and asking questions designed to exclude a physical illness (such as cancer or thyroid disease), to search for a possible genetic pattern of depression in the family tree, to define the potential contribution of alcohol or other drugs, to select the most promising antidepressant from the wide range available, to find the meaning in recent emotional traumas, and to consider whether unwieldy anger—perhaps long forgotten—seethes under cover of the ego.

Mind and body, after all, only seem disconnected. A number of studies have linked unresolved hostility to a variety of bodily illnesses, including heart attack. Injury to the brain can change not only a person's thoughts and perceptions but even his or her moral character. Could it be, then, that the use of ego defenses (see Chapter 17) can also reverberate in the body, altering brain chemistry? Might the mental process of *conversion*, responsible for Maria's burning feet, actually change the balance of norepinephrine and serotonin? Is it possible that the defense called *displacement*, which can turn a forgotten trauma into a phobia, reverberates in the network of GABA (gamma-aminobutyric acid) neurons? Might psychoanalysis itself alter the brain's chemical receptors? Does the mind—or, for that matter, the soul—exist independently of the brain, merely leaving its fingerprints on the nervous system?

Such questions, cutting to the very core of human experience, are alive in the day-to-day practice of psychiatry. They echo loudly whenever a patient like Samuel (see Chapter 6) harbors within the storm of his delirium the grief of having lost a close friend; whenever a patient like Oliver (see Chapter 1) struggles to endure, beneath blankets of intense paranoia, the agony of having lost his wife.

Remaining open to hearing and feeling the powerful story lines running through psychiatric illnesses leaves the field with one foot in the physical sciences and one foot clearly outside them. It is a stance that makes purists understandably anxious. But that is no reason to retreat from it. The validity of our perspectives and our treatments—even those that resist biomedical interpretation—must be determined by whether they alleviate patients' pain and improve their lives.

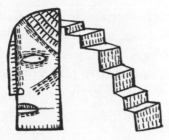

20

Psychiatric Disorders and the Mind

The mind is its own place, and in itself
Can make a Heav'n of Hell, a Hell of Heav'n.

—John Milton *Paradise Lost*

The Art of Psychiatry

The preceding chapters should leave no doubt that psychiatrists routinely draw from a number of conceptual frameworks. The theories and therapies that I will now describe, focusing more on the mind than on the brain, are among these. In the hands of skilled practitioners (and very often in combination with medications), they have demonstrated great potential to relieve many forms of human suffering.

Very few psychiatrists are expert in the use of all of these psychotherapeutic techniques (and what follows is by no means an exhaustive list). Some techniques are more anxiety-provoking for patients, whereas others are more soothing. Some therapies are relatively lengthy, taking several months or even years, whereas others are short-lived. And two patients with similar symptoms, by virtue of having different personal characteristics and life histories, may not benefit equally from any one of them.

Devising an individualized treatment strategy is one of the real arts—

and one of the greatest challenges—in the practice of psychiatry. Elements from several techniques, with or without the addition of medications, may be brought to bear. This means that the psychiatrist has both the freedom and the responsibility to pick and choose those psychiatric understandings that speak most directly to each patient's suffering.

Each man is ill in his own way.

Depression and the Mind

The core idea behind many (but not all) psychotherapies for depression is that early life experiences, generally involving disappointment, trauma or loss, have left the person psychologically vulnerable to even remotely similar stresses later in life. Self-esteem in such individuals is often quite fragile and can evaporate in the heat of failed relationships or other troubling events.

The notion that long past, perhaps even forgotten, traumas could weaken someone faced with new emotional challenges comes directly from Freud's theories about the ego and its defenses. As already discussed in Chapter 17, Freud postulated that the ego is the mind's negotiator, responsible for mediating between the instinctive drives of the id and the ethical and social constraints imposed by the superego. Faced with potentially overwhelming emotions, the ego employs protective defense mechanisms—ways of channeling and dissipating mental stress. Through the defense called *repression*, for example, unacceptable thoughts or memories could be banished into the unconscious and kept there. Through the defense called *conversion*, ideas and emotions could be changed into physical symptoms.

This process can leave the mind in delicate balance. Additional stress (such as a new reminder of an old, forgotten trauma) requires that the ego employ auxiliary defense mechanisms. The burden of this process—the increasing tension on the ego—shows up as depressed and anxious feelings.

A young man whose mother was severely ill when he was five years old, for example, might become clinically depressed when, later, upon leaving home for college, he must part with her. The separation recalls his childhood terror of abandonment and isolation. The ego, which has repressed these early emotions, must now keep a lid on them in the face of a powerful new reminder. The observable evidence of this ego tension may include symptoms of low mood, tearfulness, sleeplessness, low appetite and feelings of worthlessness.

In Toni's case (see Chapter 16), her daughter's birthday recalled her father's abusive behavior—an intense childhood disappointment. To deal with this new stress, the ego (which may have used a variety of its defenses to contain Toni's rage in the past) resorted to the defense called *turning against the self*.

Psychological approaches to depression tend either to put the patient increasingly in touch with the roots of his or her emotional pain or to alter the self-destructive thought patterns and behavior patterns that have grown from them.

Psychodynamic Psychotherapies

Insight-oriented psychodynamic psychotherapy relies on a close therapist-patient relationship, including the development of transference (see Chapter 18), as a tool to help patients identify and come to terms with the real underlying sources of their suffering. By exposing the roots of their pain, it is hoped that patients will not only experience relief from their current symptoms, but be able to chart a truer course through life in the future.

The young man on his way to college, for example, would slowly be encouraged to think and speak about his feelings when his mother fell ill and to reflect on how that early trauma might be connected to his reaction to leaving home. Moreover, the therapist might well point out manifestations of the patient's underlying fears in the therapeutic situation itself (the patient's transference). He or she might anticipate, for example, that taking a two-week vacation from practice could tap the patient's repressed feelings of abandonment and isolation—feelings that, when they occurred, could be identified, discussed and learned from.

Some insight-oriented therapies are open-ended and can be quite lengthy, whereas others are short-term and limited to between twelve and twenty sessions.

Cognitive Therapy

The cognitive model of depression hypothesizes that automatic negative thought patterns and distorted assumptions about the self lie at the heart of the illness. The patient sees the world through dark lenses that are often a legacy of disappointments, losses and traumas early in life.

Aaron Beck, the father of cognitive therapy, identified three crucial elements to the psychopathology of depression: the cognitive triad, silent assumptions and logical errors.

The *cognitive triad* refers to negative views held by depressed people about three aspects of their lives: themselves, their relationships and their futures. For example, a patient suffering with depression might see himself as inadequate, his friendships as false and his future as hopeless.

Silent assumptions, the second problem thought to underlie depression, are unspoken and inflexible conclusions people have drawn about themselves. Often, these assumptions are learned early in life through relationships with family members and peers. They may not be apparent to the patient, but a psychiatrist can find evidence of them in the consistent lessons the person takes from his or her interactions with others. An example would be the silent assumption, "If people don't like me, I can't be happy." Another example would be, "If people criticize me, it's because I'm odd."

In depression, these silent assumptions are thought to become more frequent and less realistic. A man who was unfairly and consistently criticized by his father as "a wimp," for example, may have developed the silent assumption, "If people take advantage of me it's because they sense I am weak." During a depressive period, even minor events may trigger the assumption again and again. Merely being assigned a disagreeable task at work, for example, could trigger the automatic thought, "If I weren't such a weakling, they wouldn't be doing this to me. I'm a pushover, and everyone can see it."

Logical errors, the third underlying feature of depression, constitute the cognitive fuel that propels silent assumptions. Examples include making a sweeping judgment about oneself based on a single incident, magnifying the importance of one person's opinion, or feeling responsible for events outside one's control.

Cognitive therapy seeks to make the patient aware of his or her automatic negative thought patterns, silent assumptions and logical errors. Once these have been identified, patients are encouraged to evaluate whether they are objectively true and to consider how they might have developed. The depressed man just described, for example, might be asked to review whether his assignment at work was actually given to him because he was perceived as weak. It might be, in fact, that it was a difficult task given him because of his history of producing results under unfavorable conditions—a sign of strength rather than weakness. Evidence confirming this version of what happened might be that he did the work well and was rewarded for it. It might also turn out, on reflection, that his supervisor reminded him of his father, which would be a clue to the roots of the depressive reasoning.

It is hoped that by repeatedly identifying and examining such depressive reasoning the patient will be increasingly freed from it. Patients may be asked to monitor and record their negative thoughts during the week and bring the list to the next appointment. They may also be given behavioral assignments. A man who believes all his friends have abandoned him as a worthless person, for example, may be assigned the task of calling one friend each night and writing down clear evidence supporting his assumption.

Several research studies have demonstrated that cognitive therapy is at least as successful as medication in treating patients with major depression (as long as the patients are not psychotic).

Behavioral Treatment

Behavioral theories about depression suggest that the illness begins with life stresses that jolt an individual out of his or her normal, automatic behavioral routines. This change not only leads directly to low mood, but also gives the person more unstructured time to think critically about his or her life. As mood worsens and self-criticism deepens, the person increasingly withdraws from his or her environment. Relationships begin to drift, social activities dwindle and sexual behavior is reduced. These and other lifestyle changes, in turn, further impair the person's mood, creating a "vicious cycle" that keeps the depression alive.

Treatment, which generally runs one to three months, is aimed at restoring those positive life experiences that the person has lost. Through discussion and written tests, the therapist and patient identify those things the patient finds pleasurable and others he or she finds unpleasurable. In so doing, they often come to a mutual understanding of some elements fueling the depression. A woman might, for example, have a low score for pleasurable sexual activities and a high score for stressful verbal arguments with her husband. The behaviors associated with her marriage are thereby highlighted as potential contributors to her condition.

To track the behavior-mood connection, patients are typically asked to monitor (and record) both their moods and the pleasant and unpleasant events in their lives. Doing this on a daily basis allows them to see the way their internal feelings vary with the presence or absence of pleasurable activities.

Armed with a better sense of how their behaviors are related to their depressions, patients are taught to set behavioral goals. A man who stopped his regular exercise routine after becoming depressed might set a goal of jogging one mile every other day. A depressed woman whose pleasurable phone calls to friends have ceased might set the goal of making one such call every night. One patient of mine noted how badly she felt about remaining in her bed clothes until midafternoon and set the goal of dressing every morning within forty-five minutes of waking.

Patients are advised to reward themselves when they achieve the goals they have set. My patient, for example, had decided that after one week of carrying out her dressing routine she would reward herself with dinner at her favorite restaurant. Other incentives could include buying oneself a gift, setting time aside to relax, or visiting with family.

The therapist may provide other motivations. On occasion, he or she may make continued treatment contingent on achieving certain goals. Fees might even be reduced as a reward for progress.

Sometimes patients cannot achieve their behavioral goals without being taught new personal and interpersonal skills. These could include assertiveness training, relaxation techniques or mechanisms of self-control. If a man were to report having found his job pleasurable but suddenly too stressful, he might be taught techniques of stress management that would allow him to pursue his goal of returning to work.

The patient's environment may itself contribute to his or her depression. An elderly man who has lost his wife and is living alone in an isolated area, for example, might be encouraged either to find a roommate or to move to a more populated community.

Several studies have demonstrated the effectiveness of behavioral treatment for major depression. Behavioral techniques often work very well, in fact, in depressed patients whose conditions have failed to improve despite antidepressant medications.

Interpersonal Psychotherapy

Interpersonal therapists generally agree that the symptoms of depression are sculpted by some combination of psychodynamic and biological factors. Interpersonal psychotherapy (IPT) focuses, however, on the disruptions in close social and interpersonal relationships, such as marriage, that are so often associated with the disorder. Typical disruptions include the following:

1. Prolonged or very severe grief following the loss of a loved one
2. Differing expectations between two partners in a close relationship
3. A change in one's role within a significant relationship
4. A history of inadequate and unholding interpersonal relationships, coupled with poor social skills

IPT is a short-term form of psychotherapy, generally lasting twelve to sixteen sessions. It includes an organized and detailed assessment of the workings of a patient's significant social and interpersonal bonds. When problems like those listed above are identified, patients are helped to recognize and accept the emotional pain involved, to identify nonproductive styles of communication, to devise more helpful means of being understood and to institute healing behaviors.

The official IPT manual, for example, describes a sixty-eight-year-old woman who had become depressed after losing her husband to an extended illness. Her husband's slow decline had significantly limited her life experience for years, resulting in her great unspoken anger and frustration. The manual states:

> Her symptoms included pervasive sadness and preoccupation with feelings of guilt and hopelessness. The first aim of treatment was to help the patient successfully mourn the loss, as the mourning process had been blocked by anger. The second aim was to help her to reestablish interests and relationships to substitute for what she had lost.

A second example from the manual is that of a twenty-two-year-old single man who became severely depressed one month after the breakup of his three-year relationship with his girlfriend:

> The patient, a part-time student employed as a cook, lived with his mother, who had stopped working after being hospitalized for physical problems, and subsequently, he had become depressed. Discussion of the patient's current relationships revealed that, apart from his mother, he felt close to no one.
>
> Information from the patient's past revealed a history of inadequate relationships and lack of interpersonal skills. The treatment focused on past significant relationships and on his conflicts over his relationship with his mother. The patient-therapist relationship provided a direct source of information about the patient's style of relating to others, and this information was used to modify maladaptive interpersonal patterns.

IPT has been found to be at least as effective as some antidepressants in treating the low mood, decreased work performance, decreased interests, suicidal thoughts, and feelings of guilt that so often accompany major depression. It apparently has less of an effect on depressive sleep and appetite problems and bodily aches and pains. IPT used in combination with antidepressant medication works better than either used alone.

Supportive Psychotherapy

In some cases of depression, the patient's mental energy is so compromised that psychotherapy must be limited largely to the therapist using his or her warmth, optimism and knowledge of depression to support and encourage the patient to persevere. Dr. Sidney Bloch has noted that "supportive psychotherapy" means to "carry" the patient. He has outlined its five central objectives.

1. To promote the patient's best psychological and social functioning
2. To bolster self-esteem and self-confidence
3. To make the patient aware of what can and cannot be achieved— his or her own limitations and the limitations of treatment
4. To prevent undue dependency on professional support and unnecessary hospitalizations
5. To promote the best use of available support from family and friends

Because of the tenacity of depressive thinking, hopeful messages about the great likelihood of recovery from depression may have to be repeated again and again by the therapist, lest the patient slip further into darkness.

Supportive psychotherapy is often used in conjunction with antidepressant medication. Any single antidepressant can take several weeks to work, and trials of two or more of them may be necessary before an effective one is found. During the waiting periods, supportive therapy can reduce a patient's feelings of anxiety and increase his or her level of optimism.

Mania and the Mind

Psychodynamic theorists have thought of mania as the overwrought mind's way of distancing itself from emotional pain. Using this model, the elation and feelings of omnipotence that manic patients describe can be thought of as a kind of hero's cape over feelings of vulnerability or a comedy mask over unbearable grief.

The psychoanalyst Melanie Klein believed that painful interpersonal events, including either the loss of loved ones or slavish dependency on them, were the springboard for mania. Such losses and struggles led manic patients to paradoxically disavow the need for relationships or swing to the opposite extreme of idealizing them.

In Oliver's case (see Chapter 1), the death of his wife and the impending departure of his daughter seemed to me as if they had set the stage for his manic episode.

Viewed through the lens of these theories, it is not surprising that manic patients often reject the notion that they are in any distress at all. Insight-oriented psychotherapy, which requires self-reflection, may not be useful until the mania has been treated with lithium or another medication. Even supportive psychotherapy may be limited to forging behavioral bargains with the patient that help protect him or her from physical harm, loss of relationships and financial disaster.

Schizophrenia and the Mind

There has been no shortage of controversial theories about how a person's life history might predispose him or her to developing schizophrenia. Most have centered on whether certain family dynamics may have called on patients to strike nearly impossible emotional bargains with themselves, leading to feelings of frustration and unwieldy aggression. Such conflicts include the desire to become an individual when faced with parents who cultivate dependency, the pain of choosing sides between a mother and father who are hostile to—or withdrawn from—one another, the impossible "double bind" of being encouraged to love and respect an abusive parent, and the constraints of trying to express one's true self when confined to an inflexible role within the family structure.

A few researchers have hypothesized that families most at risk of raising schizophrenic children are those including one very dominant or narcissistic parent and one very passive or dependent parent—a situation termed "marital skew." Others have focused on excessive rigidity, need for control, and coldness in parents.

These remain controversial ideas. Many families with the characteristics described above, after all, raise children free from mental illness.

As discussed in Chapter 10, a good deal of scientific data now suggest that a vulnerability to schizophrenia is inherited. If one identical twin suffers from schizophrenia, there is a 50 to 60 percent chance that the other twin will also be affected, even if the twins are raised in separate households.

Whatever the root causes, the patient's inner experience is generally regarded as one of terrifying confusion and sensory overload. The ego—the mind's negotiator—is thought to be in a constant struggle to ward off potentially destructive emotions, such as overwhelming rage. To accomplish this task, psychoanalysts believe the mind employs three major ego defenses (see Chapter 17).

One of these ego defenses is psychotic *projection*, whereby inner feelings of sexuality, hostility and chaos are irrationally attributed to others. This paints the world (a mirror of the self) as extremely dangerous and can lead to the patient being paranoid and isolative.

The second defense is *reaction formation*, which camouflages impulses or ideas that are anxiety-provoking by turning them into their opposites. A young man who was sexually abused as a child, for example, may still have the underlying desire to be close to other people. His traumatic experience, however, makes the notion of trusting and being intimate with others very threatening. Via the defense of reaction formation his inner need for relationships could be translated to an opposite and "safer" insistence on solitude.

Finally, through the ego defense of psychotic *denial*, troubling ideas, emotions and sensations can be split off from the self and experienced as hallucinatory voices or visions.

A variety of psychotherapies for schizophrenia have been explored, including insight-oriented psychotherapy and supportive psychotherapy. Although they can be extremely helpful when used by an expert in conjunction with medications, they have only a slight chance of success when used alone. One reason may be that the closeness inherent in the physician-patient relationship can be extremely threatening to schizophrenic individuals, who generally experience emotional intimacy as suffocating. The doctor, in fact, may be seen as intent on capturing the patient's soul. Another reason for the difficulties schizophrenic patients experience in therapy may be that the process leads them to project their own unspoken aggressive impulses onto the psychiatrist. In this way, an empathic doctor can be painted as hateful or evil.

The very fact that psychiatrists *do* feel and display a range of emotions may unnerve those suffering with schizophrenia. It is difficult for these patients to know for sure whether emotions are coming from inside them or belong to other people. The normal hints of anger, happiness or affection that play across a clinician's face may feel like ominous chinks in their own emotional armor.

For these reasons, psychotherapists who work with schizophrenic patients are especially attentive to and respectful of their boundaries. We know that there may be long periods of silence during sessions, as well as erratic attendance. Symptoms can evolve unpredictably.

The initial goal of therapy is to build a trusting relationship with the patient by being genuine and open, listening to the patient's pain, understanding him or her as a person (not merely a collection of symptoms), and offering advice and reassurance.

In addition to individual psychotherapy, group therapy has been used to treat schizophrenic patients for over six decades. Group members, under the direction of a therapist, help each other to express emotion, to correctly interpret the words and actions of others, to clearly convey thoughts, to generate solutions to troubling life predicaments and to form supportive relationships outside their immediate families.

Groups in which members interact freely with one another may be too stressful for patients suffering with severe psychosis. These patients are better treated in small, structured groups in which social skills and problem solving are taught through simple, straightforward lessons.

Such lessons are elements of behavioral rehabilitation. Behavioral treatments for schizophrenia focus on helping patients rebuild their social and learning skills. A patient who speaks constantly and in vivid detail about hearing voices, for example, might be encouraged to reserve that topic for his individual therapy sessions. A woman who speaks very little might be rewarded each time she appropriately joins in a group discussion. Goals of treatment might also include increasing a patient's attention span or improving a patient's grooming habits.

Finally, family therapy can be an integral part of the treatment plan for schizophrenic patients. Relatives are helped to understand schizophrenia as an illness over which the patient has little control. They may also be enlisted as partners in continuing behavioral treatments at home and in identifying and limiting those stressors that have the potential to worsen the patient's symptoms.

Phobias, Panic and the Mind

According to many psychoanalytic theorists, phobias and panic disorder begin with early impulses or traumas—for instance, "forbidden" sexual feelings toward a parent—that are distressing to the self. In order to contain them, the ego puts several of its defenses (see Chapter 17) into play. First, through *repression*, the feelings are buried in the unconscious. This alone, however, does not give the mind sufficient peace, because the buried feelings constantly threaten to blossom into conscious awareness. The ego reinforces against this through *displacement* and *projection*, a combined strategy that allows some of the fear and anxiety associated with the troubling impulses to surface, but only once they are severed from their original sources and attached to less threatening decoys.

In this way, for example, an eleven-year-old girl who becomes momentarily sexually excited while wrestling playfully with her father may *repress* her sexual feelings and later *displace* the associated fear and anxiety onto the beach where the interaction took place. But memories of that *particular* beach are still too closely linked with the anxiety-provoking episode. Therefore, the mind might *project* the fear of that beach onto the ocean itself, losing the original source of fear and anxiety like a bottle on the waves.

When this girl later seeks psychiatric care for her *simple phobia* of the ocean (which has led her to avoid all waterfront areas), part of the psychiatrist's job is to cautiously retrace the ego's steps from ocean to beach to father. In this way, psychotherapy can slowly open a safety valve, allowing the original fear and anxiety of those moments to be expressed, with a corresponding decrease in symptoms.

One could predict that in such a therapeutic process the force of *transference* (see Chapter 18) would be very much alive. The patient might, for example, unconsciously select an older male therapist and find herself attracted to him. But that therapist, if astute, would take any flirtatiousness on his patient's part not as flattery, but as a hint at the father-daughter dynamic festering beneath her symptoms.

In *panic disorder*, of course, patients report that their symptoms seem to come out of the blue, without any identifiable stressor. They may not recall being afraid of anything in particular, and may have simply been driving happily down the highway when their hearts suddenly began to race, perspiration soaked their clothing, and they felt death circling too close to bear.

This lack of identifiable stressors has fueled a view of panic disorder as primarily or exclusively biological in origin. We know, after all, that abnormalities of the thyroid or adrenal glands can cause symptoms nearly identical to those of pure panic disorder (see Chapter 12). We also know that elements of the chemical communication system, blood flow and metabolism of the brain may be abnormal in panic-prone individuals.

Yet the possibility that past experiences lie at the core of panic disorder cannot be entirely excluded. It may be that the trauma fueling panic disorder is buried more deeply than that underlying phobias. Perhaps an instantaneous memory of a past trauma, stuffed just as quickly back into the unconscious, is enough to trigger the wave of symptoms. Perhaps a deep and systematic exploration of those moments at which panic strikes would reveal unconscious environmental stressors—a billboard with an evocative image, a piece of clothing worn by a passerby, the particular time displayed on a clock. We still don't really know.

One thing we do know is that psychological treatments for both phobias and panic disorder can be extremely effective, sometimes in combination with medications and, less often, without them.

While supportive, insight-oriented and cognitive therapies have proven very helpful, a major contribution has also been made by behavior therapists. Behavioral techniques help patients with phobias to expose themselves—gradually or abruptly—to the settings or situations they fear (e.g., being in a crowd). A person with a fear of heights, for example, might first be encouraged to look out a second-story window, then to hike a small hill, then to step out onto a fifth-floor roof deck, and so on. Some of this work can be done through guided imagery, wherein the patient only imagines himself or herself in the increasingly stressful situations.

Repeatedly eliciting anxiety symptoms in this structured way often reduces or completely extinguishes them. One reason may be that the patient has learned that no terrible consequences of confronting his or her fear have actually come to pass.

Lastly, group therapy—whether supportive or insight oriented—can provide patients with hope, encouragement and an additional forum in which to voice their wishes and fears.

Obsessive-Compulsive Disorder and the Mind

The roots of obsessive-compulsive symptoms are believed by psychoanalysts to reach all the way back to childhood when new anxieties related to sexual issues prompt a child to retreat to patterns of thought and behavior typical of an earlier phase of psychosexual development (see Chapter 17).

This regression puts the child back in touch with struggles for independence and with aggressive impulses that he or she had moved beyond. Stuck amid such unwieldy drives, the mind attempts to cope primarily by using two ego defenses: *isolation* and *reaction formation*. These essentially lock up the patient's emotions and build personality traits and behavior patterns that guard against their expression. In this way, underlying aggression is encased in a character style that includes lack of emotion, passivity and ambivalence.

Aggression, however, continues to fester underground. Should life events become very stressful, the mind must contain it in some other way. It does so by redirecting mental and physical energy into obsessions and compulsions, a pathologic equivalent of "working off steam."

A boy who harbors unconscious aggressive feelings toward his father, for example, might be plagued by an obsessive thought that his father is about to fall victim to a fatal accident. The boy may worry, moreover, that simply thinking of such a tragedy actually puts his father at risk. To *undo* any potential damage his mind has done, he might feel compelled to clap his hands until they are beet red. This combination of worry and activity "distract" the boy from his true aggressive impulses.

Another example might be a young woman who is obsessed with the idea that she could harm someone if she leaves a light turned on. This might lead to a compulsive ritual wherein she checks the light switch precisely thirty times to make sure it is off. Her repetitive behavior, which is overtly protective of others, keeps her underlying wish to be hurtful under wraps.

Such psychodynamic reasoning has been challenged by biological research which suggests that obsessive-compulsive disorder (OCD) may be, in part, a bodily abnormality. The disorder is more common, for example, in patients and families struck by the neurological condition called *Tourette's syndrome*. Severe obsessions and compulsions sometimes respond to new brain surgery techniques. And a part of the brain called the *caudate nucleus* is smaller in obsessive-compulsive patients than in other people.

Many psychiatrists now think, therefore, that certain people may have a biological, perhaps inherited, predisposition to OCD that is triggered by life events.

When OCD is not severe, it can sometimes be treated successfully with insight-oriented psychotherapy (often, but not always, in combination with medications). The goal of therapy is to put the patient slowly in touch with the real drives, such as aggression, underlying his or her obsessions and compulsions. Once these are recognized and understood by the patient, the mind can relax its defenses, with a corresponding reduction in symptoms.

Psychotherapy alone is generally not effective in treating long-standing or severe obsessions and compulsions.

Behavioral techniques can be extremely helpful. These include either exposing the patient to the feared situation or preventing its associated compulsive behaviors (or both). Someone obsessed with keeping absolutely clean, for example, might be encouraged to submerge his hands in dirty water for ten minutes. The boy described above could be helped to imagine his father involved in an accident, then helped to keep his hands quietly at his sides. Such therapy is often able to extinguish the obsessive-compulsive cycle.

Posttraumatic Stress Disorder and the Mind

In posttraumatic stress disorder (PTSD) the traumatic event (or events) is quite prominent in the patient's memory, not locked away in the unconscious. The disturbing memories are so easily triggered, in fact, that the mind initially seems to cushion itself against possible reminders. It accomplishes this through symptoms such as inattention to one's surroundings, emotional numbness, social withdrawal and narrowing of one's range of thought. Patients are also at great risk of turning to alcohol or illicit drugs in order to blunt their emotions.

Eventually, however, the trauma seeps through these emotional filters, with resulting symptoms that can include sweating, nausea, disorganized thinking, flashbacks and nightmares.

Psychotherapy, often in combination with medications (see Chapter 12), can be helpful in creating a safe environment for the patient to express the fear, horror or guilt at the root of such symptoms.

A recent trauma, after all, may stir both new and old anxieties. A woman who, for example, had adopted a controlled personality style in order to contain early, troubling sexual feelings might be extraordinarily traumatized by an attempted rape. The attack could unleash a torrent of unresolved psychosexual issues that must be grappled with.

Psychiatrists treating PTSD patients attempt to carefully titrate the pace of psychotherapy to the individual. Some patients, by virtue of their underlying psychological strengths, will be able to cope with a more rapid exploration of their memories and feelings, whereas others require a very cautious, less anxiety-provoking approach.

Personality Disorders and the Mind

The ways in which psychiatrists think about patients with personality disorders provide another window on our field. For even as we acknowledge that patients with such destructive relationships and impairments in self-perception may turn out to have underlying neurochemical abnormalities (see Chapter 13), most of us do not believe that their problems will ever be fully understandable—or treatable—by virtue of our evolving knowledge of the brain. More likely, abnormal personality may be found to grow out of an unhealthy alliance of biological vulnerabilities and traumatic life events.

Psychoanalytic thinkers have viewed personality disorders as defensive strategies the mind has been forced to adopt in order to shield itself from early emotional traumas. The self thus becomes like a turtle toiling under a massive, albeit sometimes colorful, shell. This idea—that dependent, paranoid, borderline, histrionic or narcissistic people are, at core, *injured* people—fuels our empathic perspective and allows us to see beyond the troubling things they do in order to focus on the things that have been troubling to them.

When we think, for example, of Tom, Hervey Cleckley's patient (see Chapter 13), we go beyond labeling his truancy from school, stealing, cruelty to animals and repeated arrests as antisocial personality disorder. We begin to wonder what life events helped to shape his opportunism and lack of empathy. We know that a large percentage of patients with antisocial personality disorder come from economically deprived households in which parents were absent, unreliable or physically and emotionally abusive. We can conceive of Tom's mind turning the anger and disappointment of such experiences on the world. We anticipate that his apparent lack of attachment to others and disregard for the law belies inner emptiness, guilt and fear of intimacy.

In a similar way, we don't simply try to extinguish the flirtatiousness or garishness of a histrionic patient. We attempt to offer sufficient support (whether through individual or group therapy) for his or her camouflaged fear of being unlovable to surface.

Instead of merely challenging the narcissist's grandiosity, we engage that person in an empathic relationship that permits an exploration of the roots of what is actually a damaged self-concept.

Our hope is that in creating a safe enough environment, patients with any one of the personality disorders will be able to slowly let down their guards, talk about their pain, find understanding and, perhaps, outgrow the limits of their defensive shells.

Eating Disorders and the Mind

A variety of psychological theories have been proposed to explain anorexia and bulimia. Most have focused on the disorders as maladaptive forms of self-control, self-expression and symbolic hostility to which patients are driven by present or past emotional turmoil in their lives. One potential source of such stress is a parent (often a mother) who has commandeered the patient's life by treating him or her as an extension of herself, rather than a separate individual. Some theorists, in fact, see self-induced starvation or vomiting as the patient's pathologic attempt to "rid" the body of intense and unwelcome outside influences.

Other common sources of turmoil include being exposed to long-term simmering conflict between parents or being a victim of physical or sexual abuse.

When a mother and father, for example, are ambivalent about their marriage, their doubts about each other may be subtly communicated to their child. Theorists have proposed that a boy or (more commonly) a girl used as a reservoir for such feelings may perceive that his or her dependency is the only glue holding the parents together. In an unconscious effort to remain in place as the third leg of such a shaky tripod, the child might, by starving, thwart his or her development into an independent adult.

In a similar way, a young girl whose father is sexually inappropriate toward her might unconsciously attempt to control her development into a woman through the physical consequences of malnutrition, including atrophy of breast tissue and lack of menses.

Other theorists have suggested that early emotional traumas can prevent patients from developing appropriate methods of soothing themselves when they feel afraid, lonely, angry or bored. Bingeing on large amounts of food helps comfort them temporarily, but the lack of control involved eventually horrifies them and leads to self-induced vomiting.

The cornerstone of treatment for eating disorders is long-term insight-oriented and supportive psychotherapy (sometimes with medication, sometimes without). The process allows patients to vent their internal feelings and be understood as individuals with real emotions all their own. The hope is that patients can thereby "find themselves" and come to see how bottled up anger and sadness and anxiety have been fueling their disordered eating habits.

Behavioral treatments can also be helpful. These focus on the disordered eating habits themselves, rather than the emotional conflicts underlying them. A patient might be encouraged to write and sign a contract, for example, stating that he or she will consume certain quantities of food. He or she might enter a comprehensive eating disorders treatment program under an agreement to maintain a minimum body weight.

Cognitive therapy can be used to point out the faulty reasoning that drives the abnormal eating habits of many anorexic and bulimic patients. An emaciated woman who refuses to consume more than a certain number of grams of fat, for example, might be challenged to think about what consuming one extra gram would really mean. If she comes to understand that the extra gram of fat symbolizes—but isn't—a complete loss of control, she might be able to gradually relax her rigid self-control.

Family therapy can also be an important component of treatment. First, family dynamics may have set the stage for the disordered eating. Left untouched, these dynamics can perpetuate or worsen symptoms. Second, because eating disorders run in families, multiple family members may need help.

Group therapy, in which several patients meet with a group leader, can provide a relatively nonjudgmental forum for patients to share the stresses and challenges inherent in their eating disorders and in their lives in general.

Because eating disorders so often reflect issues of control, anorexic and bulimic patients tend to dislike rigidly structured therapies. They may be especially suspicious of the therapist's intentions and resolute on maintaining absolute independence. Psychiatrists must anticipate these reservations and incorporate a degree of flexibility into the therapeutic relationship.

Brain/Mind Treatment

I have been careful to point out several times in this chapter that psychotherapy is often one part of an overall treatment strategy that includes the use of medications. Scientific studies have shown that for many different psychiatric disorders, using "talk therapy" and pharmacotherapy together will very likely work better than using either alone.

The success of combining medicines aimed at the brain with psychotherapy aimed at the mind has left purists at something of a loss. The data strongly challenge any theory that explains mental illness in purely biological *or* purely psychological terms.

One explanation for the success of combined treatment is that the mind and the brain, far from being wholly separate entities, constantly affect one another. We know that damage to a person's brain, after all, can alter his or her mind to such an extent that his or her moral fiber seems changed (see the case of Phineas Gage, Chapter 9). And, in a parallel way, it may be that damage to one's psychological well-being can reverberate in the brain's network of 100 billion nerve cells, causing lasting neurological changes.

A poetic way to think about this idea is to compare the brain and the mind to a stereo speaker and the music that flows through it. A mechanical failure in the speaker can easily change harmony to dissonance. But the functioning of a perfectly good speaker also depends on the qualities of the music reaching its mechanical and electrical components. If the tones are too extreme or the volume too loud, the speaker's mechanical limitations may grossly distort the music. The speaker can even be permanently damaged.

I, and many of my colleagues, believe that psychotherapy can help bring harmony back to the music of the mind. But we also believe that without medication, certain abnormalities of the brain—whether the result of abnormal genes, of head trauma or of life's disappointments— would turn even the truest of chords to chaos. We consider ourselves physicians to the mind and the brain in equal measure.

Thinking About Society

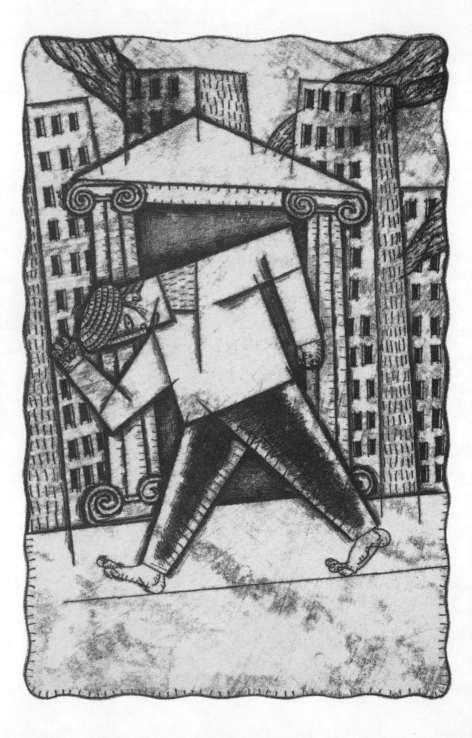

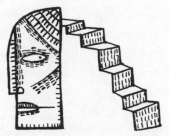

21

The Man With Nowhere to Go

I was taking overnight call covering the psychiatric emergency room of a general hospital when my beeper awakened me from a twenty-minute nap. Squinting at my watch, I saw it was just after 1 A.M. I sat at the edge of the bed half a minute, rubbed the sleep from my eyes, then walked down the hallway to the admitting nurse's desk.

The nurse handed me a consultation form on which she had written the patient's identifying information: Daniel Williams, fifty-six-year-old, divorced, homeless man complaining of depression; history of alcohol dependence, no apparent suicidal or homicidal impulses. "He's in Room 2," she said. "He says he has nowhere to go."

I started for the room. The fact that the patient had denied violent impulses surprised me. Most troubled homeless people who know the system and need help learn to claim emphatically that they are feeling suicidal or homicidal. They know that resources are so slim and hospital beds at such a premium that any psychiatric problem short of life and death usually is made to wait until an outpatient appointment is available, perhaps several days or even weeks later.

Against a constant flow of would-be inpatients, one of my roles as the

---

Portions of this chapter were first published in *The Washington Post*.

on-call physician becomes that of gatekeeper, trying to evaluate whether the suicidal or homicidal thinking a patient reports is real, attempting to defuse empty threats in order to justify keeping the ward census at a reasonable number. After nights when I have not admitted any patients, I have been congratulated by colleagues, slapped on the back and affectionately called a "wall."

But this man, I learned, was a newcomer to the emergency room; he didn't know how to manipulate the system. He had only recently lost his job, then his wife, then his home. For a month he had wandered, drinking to forget, sleeping in shelters. Tonight he had sobered up too late to secure a shelter bed, and, alone in the freezing wind, he felt his grief and exhaustion weighing more heavily than ever.

"I need to be in the hospital," he told me. "I have to get a handle on myself."

I listened at length to his description of the losses he had suffered. "Have things gotten so bad for you that you've thought of hurting yourself?" I asked.

"I would never do that," he replied.

Part of me wanted to hint at the symptoms that would justify his admission to the ward. "Some people get so angry that they start thinking of hurting someone else . . . "

"Look, Doc," he said, shaking his head, "I'm worn out. Period. I'm not mad at anyone but myself."

He denied the most serious symptoms of clinical depression or any other major mental illness. His intellect and memory were normal. He had never been admitted to a psychiatric hospital and hadn't ever been placed on medication for emotional problems. As if to offer something to reward my search for symptoms, he showed me his feet, skinned and bloody from walking the streets.

There was no question Daniel was suffering. His life had taken a turn into terrible darkness. But the health care system is still fickle about how much responsibility it will take for people whose lives are "broken" in ways that don't show up on X-rays or blood tests.

The truth is that even severe symptoms (and a lengthy history) of depression probably wouldn't have resulted in his receiving inpatient care, at least not for very long. I knew from participating in morning

rounds at similar hospitals that dangerous overcrowding and understaff-
ing meant that untreated patients routinely had to be discharged from
the ward. In my experience, these patients included many who, had
they the money or the insurance to pay for it, would have been advised
to remain in the hospital—patients with continuing symptoms of depression, who were not actively suicidal; patients who were out of touch
with reality, but not actually violent; patients with limited understanding of their medications or no easy way to renew them. It was not
unusual, in fact, for patients to be discharged after just one day.

"There's no question you need help with the problems you've talked
about," I said. "I can help you follow up with the outpatient clinic
downtown."

He took the slip of paper on which I had written the clinic address
and phone number. "I don't need to be in the hospital?" he asked,
plaintively.

"No," I said. "But I'd like to be sure you'll make an appointment with
the clinic. They may decide to schedule an admission in the future."

"I will," he nodded. He looked at me expectantly. "Where do I go now?"

Sometimes the answer to that question is simple, but not this time.
None of the shelters the night hospital staff called had any beds available. The admitting office of the hospital had no room to house another
patient on a ward. The security guard reluctantly reminded me that no
one was allowed to sleep overnight in the hospital lobby. The buses to the
airport, where homeless people have told me they sometimes find safe
corners, had stopped running. The hospital's petty cash fund had run dry.

"I can't find a place anywhere for you," I said, after nearly an hour,
shaking my head.

"It's cold," he said. "It'll be four, five hours before it's light."

I reached into the pocket of my scrubs and handed him three dollar
bills. "Maybe the subway," I suggested.

He started putting his socks over the medicated gauze I had wrapped
around his injured feet. "The subway's dangerous," he said.

I stood up. I felt frustrated, inadequate and guilty. "I wouldn't want to
be there myself," I said, extending my hand, "but there's not a lot more I
can do."

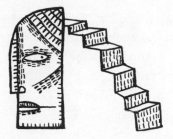

22

Psychiatry by Numbers

It is true, psychoanalysis no longer commands the attention it used to—and frankly, I think that is a good thing. We can do our work without having people breathing down our necks.

—Anna Freud

Outside Forces

When I met with Daniel early that morning, the role I could play in his life—the limits of the help I could provide him—had been partly defined by forces beyond my control. The small number of available inpatient beds, the lack of adequate shelter beds, the probable wait for outpatient services, the fact that I was tired after sixteen hours of work (with sixteen hours still to go) all reflected decisions about allocating health care resources that had been made by the hospital, the city, the state and the federal government. Daniel's clinical condition and my clinical skills were not the only factors that determined the quality of the care he received.

Daniel's case is just one dramatic example of how social values and financial concerns shape psychiatric treatment. Despite Anna Freud's optimism that the ideas that originated with her father would be allowed to branch and flower freely, the clinical practice and theoretical development of psychiatry continue to be profoundly influenced by outside agendas. These influences are at work each and every time I treat a patient, whether that person be troubled or ill, affluent or destitute.

Recognizing that psychiatric care is always colored by powerful external forces is as essential to helping patients as recognizing internal forces like transference and countertransference (see Chapter 18). It helps clinicians to think more clearly, honestly and independently about how best to restore the health and well-being of our patients.

Objective Science and the Poetry of the Mind

Psychiatry's vulnerability to outside agendas is due partly to our status as guests within the house of medicine. In medical environments, objective science holds sway. Resources flow preferentially to those specialties which offer treatments that can be shown to quickly reverse bodily abnormalities. An alcoholic patient, therefore, may have more access to medical care aimed at his diseased liver than to treatments aimed at his troubled life. The relief of suffering is most highly prized when it comes with corresponding evidence that anatomy or blood chemistry has been altered.

Many of the treatments psychiatrists offer do not pass the objective science test. We often help people get well in ways that don't show up under microscopes. Unlike finding an infection, no blood test could have traced the roots of Oliver's psychosis (see Chapter 1) to the loss of his wife. Unlike detecting a brain tumor, no CAT scan could have revealed the departure of Maria's grandson fueling her burning feet (see Chapter 4). No scientific laboratory would have turned up the terrible trauma lurking behind Toni's depression (see Chapter 16). And once these patients started to improve, no diagnostic test could have confirmed that the process of unearthing the unconscious elements of their life stories had helped them to recover—even though I felt deeply that, in each case, it had.

The fact that the workings of the mind are generally not measurable in laboratories has limited our patients' access to care and put the psychological understandings and techniques we have refined in jeopardy. Our relatively new knowledge of the brain provides a language much more tailored to (and rewarded by) the health care system. In fact, it is so much more in accord with the demands of science to speak of dopa-

mine, norepinephrine and serotonin that concepts such as the unconscious and ego defense mechanisms have become something the field
increasingly only whispers about.

The very real successes of "biological psychiatry" have led to medici-
nal cures being touted as potential cure-alls for psychiatric illness. But
the truth, as I have said before, is that our field isn't even close to
packaging mental disorders into neat biochemical bundles. We can't
explain how changes in chemical messengers in the brain change
people's lives.

Nonetheless, psychiatrists are being encouraged to abandon life story
reasoning. Because "talk therapies" are often time-consuming, medical
insurance companies (even the best ones) are structuring their pay-
ments in ways that discourage us from spending very long getting to
know our patients and encourage us to quickly prescribe them medications. A psychiatrist can be reimbursed three times as much for prescribing medicine to a different patient every fifteen minutes as he or she can
for talking to a single patient for an hour. Many insurance companies
won't pay a dime for psychiatric care unless the patient (even a patient
understandably troubled by life events) is diagnosed with a specific mental disorder. A woman who loses her job, for example, and seeks supportive psychotherapy for her low mood, anxiety and perhaps
sleeplessness might be given DSM-III-R diagnosis number 309.28, "ad-
justment disorder with mixed emotional features."

None of this is meant to diminish the tremendous contributions of
medications to reducing the suffering of psychiatric patients. Antipsychotic, mood-stabilizing and antianxiety drugs have helped countless people resume lives that had been derailed by mental illness. These
medications are critical components of the field's therapeutic armamentarium.

The trouble is that treatments aimed at the brain are so appealing to
so many factions inside and outside medicine that our other treatments
are being underestimated and underutilized. It is now entirely possible
that a patient like Toni, for example, would be admitted to psychiatric
hospitals repeatedly with recurrent major depression, tried on medication after medication, all without her history of abuse ever being uncovered. A patient like Maria might never get the opportunity to vent her
feelings about her grandson's departure.

Psychiatry's theoretical framework, which ought to remain wide enough to encompass both the brain and the mind, is now in a kind of conceptual vise. We are at risk of becoming as mechanical in our treatment of broken lives as orthopedic doctors are in their treatment of broken limbs. And it is, unfortunately, left to patients to seek out psychiatrists, clinics and hospitals that still provide the full range of understandings and treatments which they deserve. More than ever, patients need to be active, questioning and, when necessary, critical observers of their own care.

The Corrosive Role of Psychiatric Stigma

Our townsfolk were not more to blame than others; they forgot to be modest, that was all, and thought that everything was still possible for them. . . . They fancied themselves free, and no man will ever be free so long as there are pestilences.

—Albert Camus *The Plague*

The fact that the specific bodily abnormalities underlying psychiatric disorders are not fully known (and may never be) has contributed to the stigma faced by the mentally ill. For centuries, those suffering with depression, mania or schizophrenia have been viewed by many as dangerous, weak or evil, rather than ill. This allowed onlookers to consider themselves wholly different from psychiatric patients and constitutionally immune to the symptoms they exhibited.

The growth of biological psychiatry has whittled away at that kind of denial. If depression and other mental illnesses are the expression of chemical imbalances and damaged genes, after all, they can visit anyone. No one is to blame, and no one is completely protected.

Yet a large measure of the stigma associated with requiring psychiatric services remains. The evidence for this includes the shamefully low mental health coverage offered by insurance companies and the severe shortage of services provided to the homeless mentally ill. It is also apparent in the fact that those who seek supportive or insight-oriented psychotherapy in order to cope with their lives, better understand themselves or think more clearly about the future are generally not regarded by the public as introspective or health conscious, but as needy, odd or damaged. This prejudice persists in spite of the fact that people with real self-knowledge may be in a better position to give something of real value to society.

The persistence of psychiatric stigma may indicate that the public senses (correctly, in my opinion) that neurotransmitters don't tell the whole story of mental distress and illness, that life events can damage the psyche, that terrible darkness does sometimes lurk behind the symptoms of major depression, that biological psychiatry has been oversold. Yet many of these same people are not prepared to consciously entertain the real possibility that they too could harbor some similar combination of psychological and biological vulnerabilities. Tragically, they still have the need to deny the painful chapters in their own life stories by withholding compassion, understanding and resources from those who desperately need all three.

The Quiet Profession

Part of the reason psychiatry finds its conceptual base and treatment alternatives increasingly colored by social, political and economic forces (including stigma) may be that psychiatry has been locked in a kind of self-imposed silence. My colleagues and I have not given people outside the field adequate insight into what we know about the strengths *and* limitations of our work—the ambiguities, contradictions, beauty and real hope inherent in treating both the brain and the mind. It is possible, therefore, that politicians and policymakers could cut out the heart of what we do without quite knowing it.

The public still hasn't been invited to share the burden and promise of all the unanswered questions raised by patients like Oliver, Maria, Samuel, Nicholas and Toni. Yet these are crucial and far-reaching questions about the nature of human suffering, the definition of illness, the applications and limitations of scientific reasoning, the power of empathy and the proper role of psychiatry in society.

Too often psychiatrists have fantasized, like Anna Freud, that the system might accord us a kind of benign neglect, as it did for years. For decades we have naively asked to be left alone to quietly explore human thought, perception and behavior. We should have made sure, each step of the way, that we were heard.

Afterword

Having written the foregoing chapters—and read them through—I know that they answer some questions and raise many others. This is, I believe, as it should be. Too many books have offered up pat explanations of mental health and illness which, comforting as they may seem initially, ultimately fail to ring true with readers. They palpably simplify how psychiatrists think and leave the heart and wonder out of what we do.

I hope this book helps to dispel the notion that psychiatry at its best is an objective science that treats anonymous disorders. Many patients of mine have shared the same diagnosis and needed the same medications, but no two have suffered in precisely the same way or required precisely the same care. The anatomies of their illnesses have been as varied and textured as the stories of their lives.

Appendix A

DSM-III-R Diagnostic Criteria for a Major Depressive Episode and Major Depression

Diagnostic criteria for major depressive episode

Note: A "major depressive syndrome" is defined as criterion A below.

A. At least five of the following symptoms have been present during the same two-week period and represent a change from previous functioning; at least one of the symptoms is either 1) depressed mood, or 2) loss of interest or pleasure. (Do not include symptoms that are clearly due to a physical condition, mood-incongruent delusions or hallucinations, incoherence, or marked loosening of associations.)

1. Depressed mood (or can be irritable mood in children and adolescents) most of the day, nearly every day, as indicated by either subjective account or observation by others.
2. Markedly diminished interest or pleasure in all, or almost all, activities most of the day, nearly every day (as indicated by either subjective account or observation by others of apathy most of the time).
3. Significant weight loss or weight gain when not dieting (e.g., more than 5 percent of body weight in a month), or decrease or

increase in appetite nearly every day (in children, consider failure to make expected weight gains).
4. Insomnia or hypersomnia nearly every day.
5. Psychomotor agitation or retardation nearly every day (observable by others, not merely subjective feelings of restlessness or
being slowed down).
6. Fatigue or loss of energy nearly every day.
7. Feelings of worthlessness or excessive or inappropriate guilt
(which may be delusional) nearly every day (not merely self-re-
proach or guilt about being sick).
8. Diminished ability to think or concentrate, or indecisiveness, nearly
every day (either by subjective account or as observed by others).
9. Recurrent thoughts of death (not just fear of dying), recurrent
suicidal ideation without a specific plan, or a suicide attempt or a
specific plan for committing suicide.

B. 1. It cannot be established that an organic factor initiated and
maintained the disturbance.
2. The disturbance is not a normal reaction to the death of a loved
one (uncomplicated bereavement).

Note: Morbid preoccupation with worthlessness, suicidal ideation,
marked functional impairment or psychomotor retardation, or prolonged
duration suggest bereavement complicated by major depression.

C. At no time during the disturbance have there been delusions or
hallucinations for as long as two weeks in the absence of prominent
mood symptoms (i.e., before the mood symptoms developed or after
they have remitted).
D. Not superimposed on schizophrenia, schizophreniform disorder, delusional disorder, or psychotic disorder not otherwise specified
(NOS).

**Major depressive episode codes: fifth-digit code numbers and criteria
for severity of current state of bipolar disorder, depressed, or major
depression:**

1 **Mild:** Few, if any, symptoms in excess of those required to make the diagnosis, and symptoms result in only minor impairment in occupational functioning or in usual social activities or relationships with others.

2 **Moderate:** Symptoms or functional impairment between "mild" and "severe."

3 **Severe, without psychotic features:** Several symptoms in excess of those required to make the diagnosis, **and** symptoms markedly interfere with occupational functioning or with usual social activities or relationships with others.

4 **With psychotic features:** Delusions or hallucinations. If possible, **specify** whether the psychotic features are *mood-congruent* or *mood-incongruent*.

   Mood-congruent psychotic features: Delusions or hallucinations whose content is entirely consistent with the typical depressive themes of personal inadequacy, guilt, disease, death, nihilism, or deserved punishment.

   Mood-incongruent psychotic features: Delusions or hallucinations whose content does *not* involve typical depressive themes of personal inadequacy, guilt, disease, death, nihilism, or deserved punishment. Included here are such symptoms as persecutory delusions (not directly related to depressive themes), thought insertion, thought broadcasting, and delusions of control.

5 **In partial remission:** Intermediate between "in full remission" and "mild," **and** no previous dysthymia. (If major depressive episode was superimposed on dysthymia, the diagnosis of dysthymia alone is given once the full criteria for a major depressive episode are no longer met.)

6 **In full remission:** During the past six months no significant signs or symptoms of the disturbance.

0 **Unspecified.**

Specify chronic if current episode has lasted two consecutive years without a period of two months or longer during which there were no significant depressive symptoms.

Specify if current episode is **melancholic type.**

Diagnostic criteria for melancholic type

The presence of at least five of the following:

1. Loss of interest or pleasure in all, or almost all, activities.
2. Lack of reactivity to usually pleasurable stimuli (does not feel much better, even temporarily, when something good happens).
3. Depression regularly worse in the morning.
4. Early morning awakening (at least two hours before usual time of awakening).
5. Psychomotor retardation or agitation (not merely subjective complaints).
6. Significant anorexia or weight loss (e.g., more than 5 percent of body weight in a month).
7. No significant personality disturbance before first major depressive episode.
8. One or more previous major depressive episodes followed by complete, or nearly complete, recovery.
9. Previous good response to specific and adequate somatic antidepressant therapy (e.g., tricyclics, electroconvulsive therapy [ECT], monoamine oxidase inhibitor [MAOI], lithium).

Diagnostic criteria for seasonal pattern

A. There has been a regular temporal relationship between the onset of an episode of bipolar disorder (including bipolar disorder NOS) or recurrent major depression (including depressive disorder NOS) and a particular sixty-day period of the year (e.g., regular appearance of depression between the beginning of October and the end of November).

   Note: Do not include cases in which there is an obvious effect of seasonally related psychosocial stressors (e.g., regularly being unemployed every winter).

B. Full remissions (or a change from depression to mania or hypomania) also occurred within a particular sixty-day period of the year (e.g., depression disappears from mid-February to mid-April).

C. There have been at least three episodes of mood disturbance in three separate years that demonstrated the temporal seasonal relationship defined in A and B; at least two of the years were consecutive.
D. Seasonal episodes of mood disturbance, as described above, outnumbered any nonseasonal episodes of such disturbance that may have occurred by more than three to one.

Diagnostic criteria for major depression

296.2x Major depression, single episode
For fifth digit, use the major depressive episode codes (see pp. 196–197) to describe current state.

A. A single major depressive episode (see p. 195).
B. Has never had a manic episode or an unequivocal hypomanic episode.

Specify if **seasonal pattern.**

296.3x Major depression, recurrent
For fifth digit, use the major depressive episode codes (see pp. 196–197) to describe current state.

A. Two or more major depressive episodes, each separated by at least two months of return to more or less usual functioning. (If there has been a previous major depressive episode, the current episode of depression need not meet the full criteria for a major depressive episode.)
B. Has never had a manic episode or an unequivocal hypomanic episode.

Specify if **seasonal pattern.**

Appendix B

DSM-III-R Diagnostic Criteria for Manic Episode

Note: A "manic syndrome" is defined as including criteria A, B, and C below. A "hypomanic syndrome" is defined as including criteria A and B, but not C (i.e., no marked impairment).

A. A distinct period of abnormally and persistently elevated, expansive, or irritable mood.

B. During the period of mood disturbance, at least three of the following symptoms have persisted (four if the mood is only irritable) and have been present to a significant degree:

1. Inflated self-esteem or grandiosity.
2. Decreased need for sleep (e.g., feels rested after only three hours of sleep).
3. More talkative than usual or pressure to keep talking.
4. Flight of ideas or subjective experience that thoughts are racing.
5. Distractibility (i.e., attention too easily drawn to unimportant or irrelevant external stimuli).
6. Increase in goal-directed activity (either socially, at work or school, or sexually) or psychomotor agitation.
7. Excessive involvement in pleasurable activities which have a high potential for painful consequences (e.g., the person engages

201

in unrestrained buying sprees, sexual indiscretions, or foolish business investments).

C. Mood disturbance sufficiently severe to cause marked impairment in occupational functioning or in usual social activities or relationships with others, or to necessitate hospitalization to prevent harm to self or others.

D. At no time during the disturbance have there been delusions or hallucinations for as long as two weeks in the absence of prominent mood symptoms (i.e., before the mood symptoms developed or after they have remitted).

E. Not superimposed on schizophrenia, schizophreniform disorder, delusional disorder, or psychotic disorder not otherwise specified (NOS).

F. It cannot be established that an organic factor initiated and maintained the disturbance. **Note:** Somatic antidepressant treatment (e.g., drugs, ECT) that apparently precipitates a mood disturbance should not be considered an etiologic organic factor.

Manic episode codes: fifth-digit code numbers and criteria for severity of current state of bipolar disorder, manic or mixed:

1 **Mild:** Meets minimum symptom criteria for a manic episode (or almost meets symptom criteria if there has been a previous manic episode).

2 **Moderate:** Extreme increase in activity or impairment in judgment.

3 **Severe, without psychotic features:** Almost continual supervision required in order to prevent physical harm to self or others.

4 **With psychotic features:** Delusions, hallucinations, or catatonic symptoms. If possible, **specify** whether the psychotic features are *mood-congruent* or *mood-incongruent.*

Mood-congruent psychotic features: Delusions or hallucinations whose content is entirely consistent with the typical manic themes of inflated worth, power, knowledge, identity, or special relationship to a deity or famous person.

Mood-incongruent psychotic features: Either (a) or (b):

a. Delusions or hallucinations whose content does *not* involve the typical manic themes of inflated worth, power, knowledge, identity, or special relationship to a deity or famous person. Included are such symptoms as persecutory delusions (not directly related to grandiose ideas or themes), thought insertion, and delusions of being controlled.
b. Catatonic symptoms (e.g., stupor, mutism, negativism, posturing).

5 **In partial remission:** Full criteria were previously, but are not currently, met; some signs or symptoms of the disturbance have persisted.
6 **In full remission:** Full criteria were previously met, but there have been no significant signs or symptoms of the disturbance for at least six months.
0 **Unspecified.**

Appendix C

DSM-III-R Diagnostic Criteria for Somatoform Pain Disorder (307.80)

A. Preoccupation with pain for at least six months.
B. Either (1) or (2):

1. Appropriate evaluation uncovers no organic pathology or patho-physiologic mechanism (e.g., a physical disorder or the effects of injury) to account for the pain.
2. When there is related organic pathology, the complaint of pain or resulting social or occupational impairment is grossly in excess of what would be expected from the physical findings.

Appendix D

DSM-III-R Diagnostic Criteria for Delirium

A. Reduced ability to maintain attention to external stimuli (e.g., questions must be repeated because attention wanders) and to appropriately shift attention to new external stimuli (e.g., perseverates answer to a previous question).

B. Disorganized thinking, as indicated by rambling, irrelevant, or incoherent speech.

C. At least two of the following:

1. Reduced level of consciousness (e.g., difficulty keeping awake during examination).
2. Perceptual disturbances: misinterpretations, illusions, or hallucinations.
3. Disturbance of sleep-wake cycle with insomnia or daytime sleepiness.
4. Increased or decreased psychomotor activity.
5. Disorientation to time, place, or person.
6. Memory impairment (e.g., inability to learn new material, such as the names of several unrelated objects after five minutes, or to remember past events, such as history of current episode of illness).

D. Clinical features develop over a short period of time (usually hours to days) and tend to fluctuate over the course of a day.

207

E. Either (1) or (2):

1. Evidence from the history, physical examination, or laboratory
    tests of a specific organic factor (or factors) judged to be etiologi-
    cally related to the disturbance.
2. In the absence of such evidence, an etiologic organic factor can
    be presumed if the disturbance cannot be accounted for by any
    nonorganic mental disorder (e.g., manic episode accounting for
    agitation and sleep disturbance).

Appendix E

DSM-III-R Diagnostic Criteria for Schizophrenia

A. Presence of characteristic psychotic symptoms in the active phase: either (1), (2), or (3) for at least one week (unless the symptoms are successfully treated):

1. Two of the following:

   a. Delusions.
   b. Prominent hallucinations (throughout the day for several days or several times a week for several weeks, each hallucinatory experience not being limited to a few brief moments).
   c. Incoherence or marked loosening of associations.
   d. Catatonic behavior.
   e. Flat or grossly inappropriate affect.

2. Bizarre delusions (i.e., involving a phenomenon that the person's culture would regard as totally implausible, e.g., thought broadcasting, being controlled by a dead person).
3. Prominent hallucinations [as defined in (1)(b) above] of a voice with content having no apparent relation to depression or elation, or a voice keeping up a running commentary on the person's behavior or thoughts, or two or more voices conversing with each other.

B. During the course of the disturbance, functioning in such areas as work, social relations, and self-care is markedly below the highest

209

level achieved before onset of the disturbance (or, when the onset is in childhood or adolescence, failure to achieve expected level of social development).

C. Schizoaffective disorder and mood disorder with psychotic features have been ruled out. (That is, if a major depressive or manic syndrome has ever been present during an active phase of the disturbance, the total duration of all episodes of a mood syndrome has been brief relative to the total duration of the active and residual phases of the disturbance.)

D. Continuous signs of the disturbance for at least six months. The six-month period must include an active phase (of at least one week, or less if symptoms have been successfully treated) during which there were psychotic symptoms characteristic of schizophrenia (symptoms in A), with or without a prodromal or residual phase, as defined below:

Prodromal phase: A clear deterioration in functioning before the active phase of the disturbance that is not due to a disturbance in mood or to a psychoactive substance use disorder and that involves at least two of the symptoms listed below.

Residual phase: Following the active phase of the disturbance, persistence of at least two of the symptoms noted below, these not being due to a disturbance in mood or to a psychoactive substance use disorder.

Prodromal or residual symptoms:

1. Marked social isolation or withdrawal.
2. Marked impairment in role functioning as wage-earner, student, or homemaker.
3. Markedly peculiar behavior (e.g., collecting garbage, talking to self in public, hoarding food).
4. Marked impairment in personal hygiene and grooming.
5. Blunted or inappropriate affect.
6. Digressive, vague, overelaborate, or circumstantial speech, or poverty of speech, or poverty of content of speech.

7. Odd beliefs or magical thinking, influencing behavior and inconsistent with cultural norms (e.g., superstitiousness, belief in clairvoyance, telepathy, "sixth sense," "others can feel my feelings," overvalued ideas, ideas of reference).
8. Unusual perceptual experiences (e.g., recurrent illusions, sensing the presence of a force or person not actually present).
9. Marked lack of initiative, interests, or energy.

Examples: Six months of prodromal symptoms with one week of symptoms from A; no prodromal symptoms with six months of symptoms from A; no prodromal symptoms with one week of symptoms from A and six months of residual symptoms.

E. It cannot be established that an organic factor initiated and maintained the disturbance.
F. If there is a history of autistic disorder, the additional diagnosis of schizophrenia is made only if prominent delusions or hallucinations are also present.

Classification of course. The course of the disturbance is coded in the fifth digit:

1 **Subchronic:** The time from the beginning of the disturbance, when the person first began to show signs of the disturbance (including prodromal, active, and residual phases) more or less continuously, is less than two years, but at least six months.
2 **Chronic:** Same as above, but more than two years.
3 **Subchronic with acute exacerbation:** Reemergence of prominent psychotic symptoms in a person with a subchronic course who has been in the residual phase of the disturbance.
4 **Chronic with acute exacerbation:** Reemergence of prominent psychotic symptoms in a person with a chronic course who has been in the residual phase of the disturbance.
5 **Remission:** When a person with a history of schizophrenia is free of all signs of the disturbance (whether or not on medication), "in remission" should be coded. Differentiating schizophrenia in remis-

sion from no mental disorder requires consideration of overall level of functioning, length of time since the last episode of disturbance, total duration of the disturbance, and whether prophylactic treatment is being given.

0 **Unspecified.**

Appendix F

DSM-III-R Diagnostic Criteria for Bulimia Nervosa (307.51)

A. Recurrent episodes of binge eating (rapid consumption of a large amount of food in a discrete period of time).

B. A feeling of lack of control over eating behavior during the eating binges.

C. The person regularly engages in either self-induced vomiting, use of laxatives or diuretics, strict dieting or fasting, or vigorous exercise in order to prevent weight gain.

D. A minimum average of two binge-eating episodes a week for at least three months.

E. Persistent overconcern with body shape and weight.

Appendix G

DSM-III-R Diagnostic Criteria
for Anorexia Nervosa (307.10)

A. Refusal to maintain body weight over a minimal normal weight for age and height (e.g., weight loss leading to maintenance of body weight 15 percent below that expected); or failure to make expected weight gain during period of growth, leading to body weight 15 percent below that expected).

B. Intense fear of gaining weight or becoming fat, even though underweight.

C. Disturbance in the way in which one's body weight, size, or shape is experienced (e.g., the person claims to "feel fat" even when emaciated, believes that one area of the body is "too fat" even when obviously underweight).

D. In females, absence of at least three consecutive menstrual cycles when otherwise expected to occur (primary or secondary amenorrhea). (A woman is considered to have amenorrhea if her periods occur only following hormone [e.g., estrogen] administration.)

Bibliography

Ablow KR: To Wrestle With Demons: A Psychiatrist Struggles to Understand His Patients and Himself. Washington, DC, American Psychiatric Press, 1992

American Psychiatric Association: Diagnostic and Statistical Manual of Mental Disorders, 3rd Edition, Revised. Washington, DC, American Psychiatric Association, 1987

American Psychiatric Association: DSM-IV Options Book: Work in Progress. Washington, DC, American Psychiatric Association, 1991

American Psychiatric Association: Treatments of Psychiatric Disorders: A Task Force Report of the American Psychiatric Association, Vols 1–3. Washington, DC, American Psychiatric Association, 1989

Bakalar J, Baldessarini RI, Berezin MA, et al: The New Harvard Guide to Psychiatry. Edited by Nicholi AM. Cambridge, MA, Belknap Press/Harvard University Press, 1988

Bartlett: Bartlett's Familiar Quotations. Boston, MA, Little, Brown, 1980

Broyard A: Intoxicated by My Illness. New York, Clarkson Potter, 1992

Carlat DJ, Camargo CA: Review of bulimia nervosa in males. Am J Psychiatry 148:831–843, 1991

Cleghorn HM, Lee BL: Understanding and Treating Mental Illness. Toronto, Hogrefe & Huber, 1991

Cooper AM: Will neurobiology influence psychoanalysis? Am J Psychiatry 142:1395–1402, 1985

DePaulo JR, Ablow KR: How to Cope With Depression: A Complete Guide for You and Your Family. New York, Ballantine Fawcett-Crest, 1991

217

Dixon KN, Stern SL: How are depression and bulimia related? Am J Psychiatry 146:162–169, 1989

Faust D, Miner RA: The empiricist and his new clothes: DSM-III in perspective. Am J Psychiatry 143:962–971, 1986

Fava M, Copeland PM, Schweiger U, et al: Neurochemical abnormalities of anorexia nervosa. Am J Psychiatry 146:963–971, 1989

Fink PJ, Tasman A (eds): Stigma and Mental Illness. Washington, DC, American Psychiatric Press, 1992

Fitzgerald FS: The Great Gatsby. New York, Collier Books, 1986

Freud S. An Outline of Psychoanalysis (1940[1938]). New York, WW Norton, 1969

Gabbard GO: Psychodynamic Psychiatry in Clinical Practice. Washington, DC, American Psychiatric Press, 1990

Gabbard GO: Psychodynamic psychiatry in the "Decade of the Brain." Am J Psychiatry 149:991–998, 1992

Gold MS: The Good News About Panic, Anxiety and Phobias. New York, Villard Books, 1989

Goodman A: Organic unity theory: the mind-body problem revisited. Am J Psychiatry 148:553–563, 1991

Gorman JM, Liebowitz MR, Fyer AJ, et al: A neuroanatomical hypothesis for panic disorder. Am J Psychiatry 146:148–161, 1989

Grob GN: Origins of the DSM-I: a study in appearance and reality. Am J Psychiatry 148:421–431, 1991

Gunderson JG, Elliot GR: The interface between borderline personality disorder and affective disorder. Am J Psychiatry 142:277–288, 1985

Harlow JM: Recovery from the passage of an iron bar through the head. Massachusetts Medical Society Publication 2:327–346, 1868

Hollender MH, Ford CV: Dynamic Psychotherapy: An Introductory Approach. Washington, DC, American Psychiatric Press, 1990

Hyman SE, Arana GW: Handbook of Psychiatric Drug Therapy. Boston, MA, Little, Brown, 1987

Kales A, Stefänis CN, Talbott JA (eds): Recent Advances in Schizophrenia. New York, Springer, 1990

Kaplan HI, Sadock BJ (eds): Comprehensive Textbook of Psychiatry/IV, 4th Edition. Baltimore, MD, Williams & Wilkins, 1987

Kaplan HI, Sadock BJ (eds): Comprehensive Textbook of Psychiatry/V, 5th Edition. Baltimore, MD, Williams & Wilkins, 1989

Kaplan HI, Sadock BJ (eds): Pocket Handbook of Clinical Psychiatry. Baltimore, MD, Williams & Wilkins, 1990

Kendler KS, MacLean C, Neale M, et al: The genetic epidemiology of bulimia nervosa. Am J Psychiatry 148:1627–1637, 1991

Kraepelin E: Lectures on Clinical Psychiatry [3rd English Edition; authorized translation of 2nd German Edition]. Revised and edited by Johnstone T. New York, William Wood, 1917

Kuffler SW, Nicholls JG: From Neuron to Brain. Sunderland, Sinauer Associates, 1976

Lishman WA: Organic Psychiatry: The Psychological Consequences of Cerebral Disorder. Oxford, UK, Blackwell Scientific, 1987

McHugh PR, Slavney PR: The Perspectives of Psychiatry. Baltimore, MD, Johns Hopkins University Press, 1983

Mogenson GJ: The Neurobiology of Behavior: An Introduction. Hillsdale, NJ, Lawrence Erlbaum, 1977

Orwell G: 1984. New York, New American Library, 1981

Pansky B: Review of Gross Anatomy, 4th Edition. New York, Macmillan, 1979

Pato MT, Zohar J: Current Treatments of Obsessive-Compulsive Disorder. Washington, DC, American Psychiatric Press, 1991

Peck MS: People of the Lie: The Hope for Healing Human Evil. New York, Simon & Schuster, 1983

Perry S, Cooper AM, Michels R: The psychodynamic formulation: its purpose, structure, and clinical application. Am J Psychiatry 144:543–550, 1987

Pirsig RM: Lila: An Inquiry Into Morals. New York, Bantam, 1991

Rutter M: Meyerian psychobiology, personality development, and the role of life experiences. Am J Psychiatry 143:1077–1087, 1986

Sacks O: The Man Who Mistook His Wife for a Hat and Other Clinical Tales. New York, Summit Books, 1985

Sider L (ed): Introduction to Diagnostic Imaging. New York, Churchill Livingstone, 1986

Siever LJ, Davis KL: A psychobiological perspective on the personality disorders. Am J Psychiatry 148:1647–1658, 1991

Spitzer RL, Gibbon M, Skodol A, et al: DSM-III-R Casebook. Washington, DC, American Psychiatric Association, 1989

Stone EM (ed): American Psychiatric Glossary, 6th Edition. Washington, DC, American Psychiatric Association, 1988

Stunkard A: A description of eating disorders in 1932. Am J Psychiatry 147:263–268, 1990

Styron W: Darkness Visible: A Memoir of Madness. New York, Random House, 1990

Ursano RJ, Hales EH: A review of brief and individual psychotherapies. Am J Psychiatry 143:1507–1517, 1986

Vaillant GE: Adaptation to Life. Boston, MA, Little, Brown, 1977

Vaillant GE: Ego Mechanisms of Defense: A Guide for Clinicians and Researchers. Washington, DC, American Psychiatric Press, 1992

Walsh BT: Eating Behavior in Eating Disorders. Washington, DC, American Psychiatric Press, 1988

Wehr TA, Rosenthal NE: Seasonality and affective illness. Am J Psychiatry 146:829–839, 1989

Yager J, Gwirtsman HE, Edelstein CK: Special Problems in Managing Eating Disorders. Washington, DC, American Psychiatric Press, 1992

Index